Enjoy the journey

Bonnie + Adam

MW01017210

#

Aging Loved Ones

*A Guide to Organizing and
Managing the Aging Process*

B. J. Hardy, CHRP. (ret'd)
N. E. Hardy, M.A., Ph.D.

www.HardyWilsonInk.com

Hardy Wilson Ink Publishers

HardyWilsonInk Authors and Publishers, P.O. Box 28067, WestShore Centre, 2945 Jacklin Road, Victoria, British Columbia. Canada V9B 6K8

ISBN 978-0-9919331-0-5 (trade paperback)
ISBN 978-0-9919331-1-2 (electronic)

Disclaimer:
This Guide has been written to provide information to help you organize and streamline your loved one's aging process. Every effort has been made to make this Guide as complete and accurate as possible. However, there may be mistakes in typography or content. Also, this Guide contains information on accepted practices only up to the publishing date. Therefore, this document should be used as a means to capture personal information relevant to your situation. The purpose of this Guide is to educate. It is not intended to replace or supplant professional legal and/or financial advice. The authors and publisher do not warrant that the information contained in this Guide is fully complete and shall not be responsible for any errors or omissions. The authors and publisher shall have neither liability nor responsibility to any person or entity with respect to any loss or damage caused or alleged to be caused directly or indirectly by this Guide. If you do not wish to be bound by the above, please return this Guide for a full refund.

THIS BOOK

IS DEDICATED

IN

LOVING MEMORY

TO

FLORENCE EVELINE WILSON

THANK YOU FOR THE WONDERFUL MEMORIES

IT WAS AN AMAZING JOURNEY.

Contents

Acknowledgements

Few projects are ever completed in isolation and this book is no exception. We are grateful for the contribution and ongoing support of family, friends, and professionals working in related fields. Specifically, we wish to thank those who shared their professional expertise, insights and wisdom:

Linda Devoir Ames

Elizabeth Hardy Backer, RMT, LPN

Loretta K. Bosma, BSW, RSW

Beverley Fitzsimonds, RN, NM

Virginia Pike Gielow

Richard W. Hardy, B.A.

David Meir, M.B., Ch.B., D.C.H.

Jennifer L. Rudolph, B.A., M.A.

Jill Garland Wilson, RT.

Susan D Zimmerman

A special thank you is given to C. Lynn Jordan, our Publishing Consultant, for her support, expertise, and patience.

The cover picture was produced by Susan and Peter Zimmerman with the able assistance of Mona Smith.

Note to the Reader

To facilitate the completion of the relevant information sheets, a complete downloadable package is available from our website: www.HardyWilsonInk.com.

Not all Information Sheets will be relevant to your situation at this time. However, you may find them useful as aging progresses.

Please note these are copyrighted materials and are made available to the purchasers of this book.

Introduction

I will never be an old man. To me, old age is always 15 years older than I am.

Bernard M. Baruch (1870 - 1965)

Welcome to Aging Loved Ones: A Guide to Organizing and Managing the Aging Process. Through no fault, will, or planning of your own, you have lived through some of the most wonderful discoveries and creations in the history of mankind.

You are surrounded by things that are automatic, super-sonic, self-directed, and self-perpetuating. You accept as your due the promises of more flexible bodies, younger skin, longer lasting beauty. There are pills to prevent, minimize and/or cure just about any disease you could discover while exploring the Internet. Science and knowledge are at your fingertips - you can access, download, preserve and/or delete more communications in a day than your ancestors experienced in a lifetime. Whether history will report that you are indeed living better than previous generations, it is a fact that you are living longer.

1

Increased longevity provides you with opportunities to stretch your imagination explore your talents and enjoy your passions well into your 'golden years'. While you reap the benefits and joys of longer life, you also face the challenge of witnessing the impact of the aging process on your parents or other loved ones.

AUTHORS' NOTE: *Within this Guide the term parent(s) has been used as a universal term to encompass any aging loved one(s).*

At a time when you're beginning to acknowledge the first hints of personal limitation, your parents seem to require more of your time and energy just to cope with the basics of living.

A few decades or so ago, people started talking about the 'Sandwich Generation', a name generously given to those approaching the threshold of the promised 'golden years' only to find they were not alone. Trailing behind, hanging on to a rather familiar chord, were the adult children. Up ahead, becoming clearer every minute was the smiling face of Mom, Dad, an older friend or a partner.

Even as you recognize that your energy banks are finite, you are being called upon to minimize the impact of aging on your parent(s). Your grandchildren crave your attention and your adult children still need your help as they move through the maze of life. Some days life feels like you're living in a sandwich and beginning to ooze around the edges. If, in fact, there is only so much energy to go around, then it would be wise for you to plan ways to make the most of what you have. This Guide is designed to help you with that planning.

It is intended to:

- ease and simplify the process of assisting your parent(s) through the transitions of aging.
- examine the signs that may indicate loss of physical, mental and/or emotional abilities
- explore a variety of options available to minimize or compensate for diminished capacity.
- identify short and long term care options and the concept of aging in place.
- assist with the development of a flexible care plan for your parent, and
- identify and organize information pertinent to your parent's care.

This is your Guide; make it work for you. Throughout each section, you will have the opportunity to record facts and thoughts unique to your parent's (and your) situation. This personalized Guide will serve as a valuable resource and, as well, provide a format for strategically planning future actions.

Aging is a process. The key to creating a progressive strategy, designed to work for both you and your parent, is to begin planning as soon as possible. You are fortunate if your parent is in good health, coping well with daily living, and enjoying all that life has to offer. Whether this is the case or not, now is the time to take a forward look. Begin to accumulate the information you will need at your fingertips as the aging process continues. Use the information sheets included within this Guide to assemble, coordinate and maintain all pertinent information in one place.

AUTHORS' NOTE: *Not all Information Sheets will be relevant to your situation at this time. However, you may find them useful as aging progresses.*

Watching a loved-one age can be a frustrating and difficult time. It is the purpose of this Guide to help you organize and simplify the process, leaving you and your parent(s) free to enjoy a peaceful and hassle-free transition together.

Following is a Personal Data sheet to be completed either with your parent(s) or on their behalf. It will help you begin the process of capturing details, and relevant contact information that may be needed in future. You may also want to make copies of legal documents such as birth certificates, driver's license, passports, medical cards, Social Insurance or Social Security Numbers, etc., and note on these sheets where the originals and copies are stored or filed.

Personal Data Worksheet

Parent's Full Name_____

Date of Birth _____Certificate Number_____

Country_____State/Province_____ City_____

Social Insurance/Security Number_____Blood Type:_____

Driver's License Number_____Expiry Date_____

Passport Number_____Expiry Date_____

Health Related Information

Allergies/Sensitivities

Foods

_____
_____
_____

Drugs

_____
_____
_____

Other

_____
_____
_____
_____

Permanent Address or Facility Contact Information

_____
Facility Name

Street Address_____

Apt. No._____

City_____ State/Province_____

ZIP/Postal Code _____

Telephone _____ Cell Number _____

E mail_____ Web Address _____

Emergency Contact Numbers

Family

Name_____ Number_____

Name_____ Number_____

Name_____ Number_____

Name_____ Number_____

Friends

Name_____ Number_____

Name_____ Number_____

Name_____ Number_____

Name_____ Number_____

Neighbors

Name_____ Number_____

Name_____ Number_____

Name_____ Number_____

Name_____ Number_____

7

Affiliations

Religious_____ Contact Name_____

Contact Number(s) _____ _____

Memberships_____ Contact Name_____

Contact Number(s) _____ _____

Social Activities/Groups

Contact Name_____

Contact Number_____

Contact Name_____

Contact Number_____

Contact Name_____

Contact Number_____

Friends (Names and Addresses or Place Where Information Stored):

Name   Address   Phone

_____   _____   _____

_____   _____   _____

_____   _____   _____

_____   _____   _____

Information also available:
in address book☐; on CD☐; on computer☐;elsewhere☐;_____

Other Relevant Information

_____

_____

_____

_____

_____

Perceptions and Expectations

Origins are of the greatest importance. We are almost reconciled to having a cold when we remember where we caught it.

Marie von Ebener-Eschenbach

Before we explore the strategies to help us manage an aging parent, spouse or friend, it may be prudent to create a base line or foundation from which we can proceed.

Seniors today, are often promoted as vibrant and active people pursuing goals and activities that fulfil their dreams. It hasn't always been so.

History, literature, even some old movies portray the life of the elderly as one of loneliness, abandonment and often poverty and neglect. Water cooler conversations chuckle over stories of the shuffling, slow gait of a heavily clothed old man. These same people express annoyance and even anger as a senior-driven scooter blows by them on the sidewalk with horn blaring. Then there's the portrayal of 'The Home', a dingy, cold, Spartan place where folks who can no longer live on their own are placed to exist until the end of their days. Personal space is limited to a small bed, one of four jammed into an airless room. Only a faint ray of setting sun sneaks through the high sealed window to mark the passing of another day.

An over dramatization? Perhaps. There are, however, elderly folks who have been 'warehoused' by their families; put into the care of others and all but forgotten. A signed-over pension check and the odd gift or card on special occasions is all the support given to these veterans of life.

Embarrassment at the behaviors and antics of the elderly often turns to mimicry and comic relief. Some of these behaviors have nothing to do with aging but with the individual personalities of those 'acting up'.

It is vitally important to recognize a change in behavior that may reflect the impact of aging. There is a wide range of ways to support and relieve the burden of aging, each explored in other sections of this Guide.

It is also vital to keep your sense of humor as you begin the journey of caring for your aging parent. Laugh with your parent, not at them.

Criticism, ridicule, annoyance and vindictiveness have no place in this process. In fact, surrounding your parent with negative emotions even when none are present will significantly impair your ability to perform the many tasks needed to establish and maintain the process of managing your parent.

At the end of this section, there are questionnaires designed to help you work through overt and often hidden expectations and motivations you may have of the elderly. Think through these questions. Are there 'triggers' that evoke negative responses to your parent; to their aging; to the added responsibility of making their journey as comfortable as possible? If so, then this is the time to think about your coping strategies, your responses and how to work with, around or through them.

We perceive the world around us through a number of filters, not the least of which is our own expectations. We begin most days with an understanding of how the hours will unfold. We accept that our routine will lead us where it usually does. We draw on skills and talents, as we always have, to achieve predictable results. We may choose to enhance or upgrade those skills; however, that process will also fit our expectations.

We often see, hear, and feel what years of experience tell us to expect. Your parent is the composite of decades of experience and subsequent learned responses. They have lived through and survived the challenges and joys of a life only briefly shared with you. Their perception of today's world has to differ from yours, as must their expectations.

Your parent is also the product of his/her family of origin – the unique group of people into whom s/he was born. This is where your parent first learned about relationships, responsibilities, religious beliefs, and work ethics. It is here, within this family unit, that your parent developed values and a moral code that provide the foundation of the life they chose to live.

This composite of how life was lived is what they brought to your family of origin. Patterns, habits, even mannerisms became part of the air you breathed as a child and later accepted as an adult. Consider the questions outlined at the end of this section. Talk with your siblings and, if possible, with your parent's siblings. Enjoy this time of exploration as you delve into what made your parent who and what s/he is today and equally as important, what made you who and what you are. Use this as a base line only, knowing that behaviors, attitudes, perceptions can and do change as we evolve.

Life-long responses to circumstances and situations may not have served your parent as well as you would like. However, they developed approaches and strategies for coping and meeting their specific needs. Over the years, these coping responses formed their habits. As with all habitual responses, those that appear to work best for us become the foundation upon which we base our concept of internal comfort and external security.

It is very likely that compromising this sense of comfort and security will be met with resistance. As the limitations of advancing age are felt, it is more likely that your parents' behaviors will become further entrenched in an effort to maintain familiar patterns. These will not easily be given up just because there is external pressure trying to impose different standards or patterns of behavior *for your own good'*. (Especially when this pressure comes from a child they have raised, and they have always been the ones who decided what constituted good for the welfare of that child.)

So, what's the situation here? We have a man or woman whose independent lifestyle is being threatened by physical and/or mental limitations. Often, with this realization, comes the fear of losing control, not just of decisions and choices, but of the body and mind as well. Learned responses and routines are being challenged.

On the other hand, we have a post-fifty adult looking forward to reaping the benefits and freedoms of retirement. The Golden Years beckon, offering the realization of dreams held during the child rearing and employment years. Yet, the added responsibility of assisting a loved-one to handle the transitions brought on by aging is becoming a reality for many middle aged adults. As the parent's physical and mental capacity diminishes, the resources needed to support and care for them increases.

REMEMBER: *If you always do what you've always done, you'll always get what you've always got.*

Witnessing the decline of a loved-one elicits a plethora of emotions. One less recognized is the fear arising from this glimpse into our own future. With the twinges of middle age evolving into aches and discomfort, it isn't difficult to understand the frustration and exhaustion inherent in accepting our evolving relationship with a parent.

Diminished capacity, together with inherent limitations, both physical and mental, places a definite strain on family relationships. Obviously, the relationship between the parent and adult child caregiver begins to reverse, and interactions with other family members can become confused and troubled. It is not unusual for relatives, especially those who live away from the parent, to place unfair

14

expectations on the caregiver sibling. Protected from direct involvement by distance, they often sit in judgment or back off altogether. It is important that the primary caregiver be given the support and understanding of all family members. To encourage this, you will want to include your siblings, as well as your parent(s), in as many decisions as reasonable. Email can greatly facilitate this process through simultaneous interaction with several family members. Decisions can be made in a timely manner and conflict minimized.

> **CAUTION:** *E-mail often eliminates the most effective communication tool, that of body language. Choose your words carefully and stick to the facts with as little editorial or judgmental comment as possible.*

Gaps in family relationships often widen when written communication is misunderstood or misinterpreted. Clarity is essential in order to get a message across as a-emotional information.

The following Information Sheets are designed to help you identify customs, attitudes or beliefs you hold that may impact the way you view and/or care for your aging parent. The roles assumed by your parent as you were growing up may now need to be transferred to another. The role(s) you have or have not assumed within your own family may also need to be revisited in light of your parent's increasing limitations.

Over the years, you and your parent have developed an adult-adult relationship, however, there may be 'old baggage' from years gone by that easily become 'triggers' or 'buttons' that, when pushed, cause a series of negative emotions and/or responses in either of you. It is important, if possible, to identify such 'buttons' or 'triggers' and to think about ways to address the 'old baggage' so that it no longer causes pain in one another. If this doesn't appear to be possible, then you may wish to devise a strategy to avoid touching on subjects guaranteed to elicit anger, bitterness or guilt. Hopefully, working through these Information Sheets, will help you address some of these issues.

AUTHORS' NOTE: *In case you are at a loss for appropriate descriptive words to categorize yourself, or your parent, a list of non-threatening words has been included with the Information Sheets at the end of this Section.*

Family of Origin Responsibility Chart

PERCEPTIONS AND EXPECTATIONS
Family of Origin Responsibility Chart©

	Mother	Father	You	Sibling(s)	Other (Specify)	N/A
Household						
Transportation						
Legal						
Financial/Investment /Taxes						
Medical						
Social Activities						
Vacation Plans						
Education						
Spiritual/Religious						
Community						
Special Holidays						
Pets/Care						
School Activities/ Involvement						
Hobbies/Activities						
Recreational/Sports Activities						

When you lived at home, as a child, teenager, and young adult, who assumed responsibility for, and made the decisions impacting, the following? (*Check any that apply; check **all** if the family made collaborative decisions*).

17

Perceptions and Expectations Questionnaire

Family Roles and Interactions

1. In relation to other siblings, where were you placed in your family?

   Only Child__ Eldest__ Youngest__ Middle____

2. What impact did this placement have on you then and now?

   _____
   _____
   _____
   _____

3. What role did you play in your family of origin?

   _____
   _____
   _____
   _____

4. What words would you choose to describe your relationship with folks a generation older than your parents?

   _____
   _____
   _____
   _____

5. What role did grandparents play in your family?

_____

_____

_____

_____

6. How were *your grandparents* perceived

(a) by your parents?

_____

_____

_____

_____

(b) by you and your siblings?

_____

_____

_____

_____

7. How were the *grandparents of your peers* perceived by you and your siblings?

_____

_____

_____

_____

8. Where did your grandparents live prior to their deaths?

On their Own _____

With Family _____

On their Own with External Help _____

Assisted Living _____

Full Care _____

9. (a). What is the norm in your culture for housing of elders?

On their Own _____

With Family _____

On their Own with External Help _____

Assisted Living (external) _____

Full Care (external) _____

(b). Is this appropriate/acceptable for you?

_____

Your Parent(s)?

_____

Perceptions and Expectations Questionnaire

Personal Perceptions

1. When you envision an elderly person, what words come to mind?

    _____   _____
    _____   _____
    _____   _____

2. What words would a stranger use to describe your parent(s)?

    _____   _____
    _____   _____
    _____   _____

3. What words would you use to describe your parent(s)?

    _____   _____
    _____   _____
    _____   _____

4. (a) How would a casual acquaintance describe you?

    _____   _____
    _____   _____
    _____   _____

21

(b) What words would your parent(s) use to describe you?

_____   _____

_____   _____

_____   _____

(c) Is there a difference? Why?

_____

_____

_____

_____

5.   (a) Identify patterns of 'emotional blackmail' or 'buttons' that your parents use when interacting with you.

_____

_____

_____

_____

(b) Identify patterns of 'emotional blackmail' or 'buttons' that you use when interacting with your parent(s).

_____

_____

_____

_____

6. What behavior can you develop to minimize the negative impact of these triggers on you and on your parent(s)?

_____

_____

_____

_____

Word List

Academic	Confident	Expressive
Accurate	Confused	Extroverted
Adventurous	Conscientious	Exuberant
Aggressive	Considerate	Fearful
Agreeable	Contented	Firm
Amiable	Controlled	Forceful
Animated	Conventional	Friendly
Antagonistic	Convincing	Frivolous
Anxious	Cooperative	Funny
Appealing	Cynical	Fussy
Argumentative	Daring	Generous
Assertive	Decisive	Gentle
Astute	Demanding	Good-mixer
Attractive	Dependable	Good-natured
Bold	Determined	Greedy
Brave	Devious	Gregarious
Calm	Diplomatic	Grumpy
Cantankerous	Direct	Happy
Captivating	Disciplined	Healthy
Careful	Dishonest	Helpful
Caring	Dominant	High-spirited
Caustic	Domineering	Honest
Cautious	Dynamic	Hostile
Charming	Eager	Humble
Cheap	Easy-going	Humorous
Cheerful	Effective	Impartial
Competitive	Efficient	Impatient
Compliant	Enthusiastic	Impulsive
Complicated	Even-tempered	Independent

Insightful	Parsimonious	Self-reliant
Insistent	Patient	Sensitive
Inspiring	Peaceful	Sickly
Introspective	Perceptive	Simplistic
Introverted	Persistent	Slovenly
Irresponsible	Persuasive	Sociable
Irritating	Petty	Soft-spoken
Jovial	Pioneering	Spiritual
Joyful	Playful	Stimulating
Kind	Poised	Strong-willed
Lazy	Pompous	Stubborn
Lenient	Practical	Submissive
Light-hearted	Precise	Surly
Logical	Predictable	Sympathetic
Loyal	Private	Systematic
Magnanimous	Provocative	Tactful
Magnetic	Puny	Talkative
Maudlin	Refined	Thorough
Moderate	Reserved	Tidy
Modest	Respectful	Timid
Muddled	Responsible	Tranquil
Neat	Responsive	Tyrannical
Needy	Restless	Unrealistic
Neighborly	Robust	Vigorous
Obedient	Rude	Violent
Obliging	Sacrificing	Willing
Observant	Sanctimonious	
Optimistic	Sarcastic	
Original	Satisfied	
Out-going	Self-focused	
Outspoken	Selfish	

This Thing Called Independence

Old Age is like everything else. To make a success of it you've got start young.

Fred Astaire

What is this thing called independence? We value it in our own lives, encourage its development in our children, praise and respect those countries and organizations that support it, yet take it for granted and assume it will always be an option. Dictionaries suggest many definitions including:

- Freedom from reliance on, or control by, others
- Self-subsistence or maintenance
- Direction of one's own affairs without interference
- Thinking for oneself
- Self-directed.

The concept of living independently is subject to personal interpretation. It does not mean the same for everyone nor is it valued by all to the same extent. What does it look like to your loved one? What does it mean to you? Is there a difference? By what criteria will you measure your parent's ability to remain independent? For some, independence has always been a way of life. Some made choices that encouraged dependence on others - spouses, family, and government systems. However, there comes a time for all of us, when activities we have taken for granted, may not be a part of our daily routine. Our ability to live life as we choose may be changing. Many elderly folks feel independence gradually slipping away with advancing years and take steps to camouflage or compensate for it as situations necessitate. Others are surprised and/or aggravated when limitation complicates or prevents them from performing routine tasks. Some stubbornly 'dig in their heels' and fight or simply ignore situations that might threaten their loss of control over their own lives.

Changes may be subtle at first. The loss of dexterity, buttons that can no longer be managed, lids that can't be loosened, or the inability to pick a fallen item off the floor, may, at first, simply cause minor frustrations. Misplaced keys, skipped appointments, or changes in personal hygiene, may be overlooked as momentary forgetfulness. Memory lapses, disorientation, confusion around medications, or increasing incontinence, however, are causes for a more significant concern.

In order to identify changes to regular behavior patterns, it is necessary to know what normal or usual activity looks like. Has your parent always been particular about appearance and personal hygiene? Did your loved one always maintain a regular schedule of medical, dental, and personal care appointments? Has that changed? Do they have a history of taking prescription medication or natural supplements as part of their regular routine? Or, do they spurn professional advice and instruction in favor of what their neighbor or favorite columnist recommends?

CAUTION: *Be aware that some couples will cover for one another's limitations. It is only when one becomes seriously ill or dies that family members discover how much the well-being of the survivor has deteriorated.*

At the end of this section, you will have an opportunity to establish a behavior baseline for your parent(s). If you have not had occasion to observe your parent during recent years, you may want to solicit input from close friends, other family members, as well as your parent. Keeping these information gathering sessions as light and unobtrusive as possible, can minimize the inference that something is wrong. Knowing what information you need before interacting with your parent or external sources, will make it easier to frame questions as part of normal conversation.

Once you have created a behavior baseline, it is important to identify how you will know your parent is deviating from normal activity. You may want to think about and record what 'warning' signs will indicate that established patterns are changing and what options are available to lessen or close the gap between normal behavior and these changes.

The involvement of your parent(s) in discussions about the potential transition from independence (as they define it) to the relinquishing of control over specific activities, will contribute significantly to the success of this process.

Quite often, these conversations don't begin until immediately before or soon after a significant moment or crisis, such as:

- Death or permanent hospitalization of the spouse, partner or close friend
- A fall resulting in permanent physical or emotional trauma
- Onset of disease or injury resulting in limited capability or disability
- Need for life-supporting medications.

How much better it would be if the subject of possible social, physical and/or mental limitations could be discussed before changes were imminent. As well, now is the time for discussions around how your parent views the future unfolding. What are their concerns, wishes, suggestions? If all things remain equal, how do they want to live out their lives? You may be surprised to learn that your loved one has given considerable thought to this. On the other hand, you may meet with resistance born of fear and/or lack of interest, the sense that there will be lots of time to think about such dark things. In any event, you will need to prompt such discussions either informally, as you chat about what's happening in the lives of friends or other family members, or in a more formal and structured manner. You know your parent and the format that will best suit their communication style.

> **CAUTION:** *Proceed slowly. Be aware of defensive body language (in both of you) and strive for a more comfortable interaction. Paraphrase words, situations or suggestions in non-threatening language. Know what you need before you begin to casually 'probe' for information. If you can, tie your discussion to events happening in your parent's social circle. 'I wonder what Marge will do now that George is dead' or 'how did Ruth know it was time to sell her house?' or 'how does Dennis like his new*

retirement home?' You can ask for clarification if you truly don't understand the implications of what's being said, however, don't push. Use open-ended questions to encourage your parent's comfort with sharing. Unless there's a pressing need for action, enjoy the luxury of spreading these conversations over leisurely periods of time.

The establishment of regular appointments with an optometrist and audiologist will ensure that changes in hearing and visual acuity will be diagnosed early. Please note that large print books may compensate for failing eyesight, however, large print magazines will offer advertising specific to the seniors market. You may wish to screen this reading material accordingly.

The following section provides considerable information on various options available to help independent seniors live safely and comfortably. You will have an opportunity to complete a list of local services, contact numbers, and other pertinent details specific to your parent's current and potential needs. Before you move on, take some time to consider your parent's understanding and appreciation of independence. Review the checklists included with this section and personalize them according to your/your parent's preferences

It is important for you (and your parent if possible) to identify what 'independence' means for your parent. Is it simply continuing to live where and as they have always lived? Is it the freedom to make choices and decisions free of interference from others? If so, how do they define interference? Is it different from needing help now and then or delegating specific tasks to external sources? How willing are they to supplement or complement their independence when abilities become limited? How will you/they know when external resources are needed?

Once you are clear on how your parent views the process of aging, and you have discussed various options to ensure s/he lives safely and well, you can begin the process of identifying behaviors and attitudes that might indicate the need for supplemental help.

CAUTION: *It is so important to have these discussions well before your parent's faculties begin to fail. The ultimate goal is for future transitions to be seamless and comfortable for all concerned - especially for your parent. They need to feel in control of decisions impacting their life. Try to encourage an atmosphere of partnership during your chats or the feeling of 'we're in this together', as indeed you are. It will*

33

go a long way to forming a comfortable base from which you both are able to introduce changes to compensate for declining ability.

As you explore the various responsibilities and tasks that make up your parent's daily life, there will be some that are considered their sacred domain. Control over other activities, however, could be relinquished with little or no regret at all.

The following Record of Change Chart© is intended to give you an insight into both subtle and dramatic changes which are taking place as a direct result of aging. It may be that activities which seem normal to a young person have become completely foreign to the elderly. For instance, as a working adult, you may shower every morning, and again after exercise. An elderly person may believe it sufficient to shower twice weekly. When filling out the sheet, under bath/shower normal you might write twice weekly. A subtle change might be a reduction to once per week, and a warning sign might be refusing to bathe more than monthly. Similarly, under Social Activities: Groups, a weekly Bridge Game might be classified as normal especially if the person has been doing it for many years. A declining interest in weekly games may indicate a subtle change associated with reduced energy, or the need to retire early. However, a sudden withdrawal from the weekly game and a total cessation of participation may be a warning sign of change in the ability to concentrate, or of memory loss. Alternatively, it may be less sinister, and may be associated with the passing of a long term table partner, hence a change in the social nature of the game. Either way, such a change warrants further exploration.

Once changes have been identified, it is imperative that decisions regarding follow-up actions be made. Thus, the 'Closing the Gap Action Sheet©' should be completed. If you have recognized changes, no matter how subtle, write Yes, or simply Y in the appropriate box in the first column. At this point a decision should be made as to what actions must be taken, if any. This decision may involve only you, you and your parent, you, your parent and your siblings, or you, your parent and professional advisors and caregivers. Any given situation may require no action be taken at the time, but may be an indicator of the need for future action.

Record of Change Information Sheet

THIS THING CALLED INDEPENDENCE
Record Of Change©

Behavior	Normal	Subtle Changes	Warning Signs
Personal Hygiene			
Face/Hands			
Bath/Shower			
Finger/Toe Nails			
Make-up			
Toilet Routine			
Daily Routine			
Meals			
Preparation			
Eating Habits			
Nutrition/ Hydration			
Medications			
Correct Doses			
Timeliness			
Sleep Activities			
Naps			
Exercise			
Group			
Alone			

THIS THING CALLED INDEPENDENCE
Record Of Change©

Behavior	Normal	Subtle Changes	Warning Signs
Social Activities			
Friends/Family			
Phone			
Write			
Visit			
Group(s)			
Weekly Routines			
Mental Activities			
Mind Stimulation			
Puzzles & Games			
Reading			
Writing			
Personal Journal			
Cards Letters			
Business			
Bill Payments			
Insurance Claims			
Income Tax Submissions			

37

THIS THING CALLED INDEPENDENCE
Record Of Change©

Behavior	Normal	Subtle Changes	Warning Signs
Memory			
Activities			
Appointments			
Personal Dates			
Regular commitments			
Current Events			
Recent Past			
Decades Ago			

Closing the Gap Action Sheet

THIS THING CALLED INDEPENDENCE
Closing The Gap Action Sheet©

Behavior	Changes Identified Yes/No	Actions Taken or To Be Taken
Personal Hygiene		
Face/Hands		
Bath/Shower		
Finger/Toe Nails		
Make-up		
Toilet Routine		
Daily Routine		
Meals		
Preparation		
Eating Habits		
Nutrition/ Hydration		
Medications		
Correct Doses		
Timeliness		
Sleep Activities		
Nightly		
Naps		
Exercise		
Group		
Alone		

THIS THING CALLED INDEPENDENCE
Closing The Gap Action Sheet©

Behavior	Changes Identified Yes/No	Actions Taken or To Be Taken
Social Activities		
Friends/Family		
Phone		
Write		
Visit		
Group Activities		
Weekly Routines		
Mental Activities		
Mind Stimulation		
Puzzles & Games		
Reading		
Writing		
Personal Journal		
Cards Letters		
Business		
Bill Payments		
Insurance Claims		
Income Tax Submissions		

THIS THING CALLED INDEPENDENCE
Closing The Gap Action Sheet©

Behavior	Changes Identified Yes/No	Actions Taken or To Be Taken
Memory		
Activities		
Appointments		
Personal Dates		
Regular commitments		
Current Events		
Recent Past		
Decades Ago		

41

Legal and Financial Management

A table, a chair, a bowl of fruit and a violin;
what else does a man need to be happy?

Albert Einstein

It is important to stress, as has been done in previous sections of this book, the benefits to establishing, as early as possible an on-going conversation with your parent about their current and future abilities, health and mental acuity. Collaborating and exchanging opinions and suggestions with your parent will help to build mutual trust as they anticipate losing potential power and control over their own activities.

With legal and financial considerations and/or changes, it is not only recommended but is essential that affairs be put in order while your parent is still able, alert and aware of what s/he is signing.

Each decade brings with it new experiences, some challenges and often a few limitations. Ten years can make a significant difference as we begin to age. In fact, a very few years can change our mobility, compromise our memory, and greatly limit our ability to make legal decisions and choices.

How can you best support your parent during this time of transition? Begin by examining the end and working backwards to the present time.

Most parents will have prepared a will at some time during their lives, wanting to ensure that all they worked for was passed on to the next generation. Years ago it was accepted that beneficiaries of life insurance instruments would receive their money long before the will was probated and fees were paid for legal, accounting and government services. Often, when bequests were finally received, they were considerably less than either the writer of the Will or the beneficiary had expected.

There are a few uncomplicated steps that could help you avoid lengthy delays and expensive costs associated with the management and ultimately the disposition of your parent's assets. You will find a series of work sheets at the end of this section. Use these to prompt discussions about simplifying your parent's life as well as your own. It is hoped that you are approaching these discussions without a sense of urgency and can allow ample time for your parent to gain a sense of comfort with the processes.

Step One: Establish a Current Will with Living Beneficiaries

How current is your parent's will? Are the executors still alive and willing to perform this service? Are the beneficiaries current? Have there been deaths, births, or other changes (financial, personal, or property) that may require further consideration? Was the most recent will drawn up on a form purchased on-line, at a stationery store or by a lawyer?

The first step in helping your parent manage their finances is to insure that s/he has a current legal will prepared by a lawyer (avoids potential claims of influence) that appoints non-professional executor(s). Why appoint a non-professional executor? Appointing a banker, accountant, lawyer, etc., to be executor(s) will most often generate considerable costs and may delay the disposition of assets. If it is not feasible or advisable for your parent to appoint one or more of his/her beneficiaries or trusted friend(s), then it is important to know potential costs and processes at the time the will is prepared.

You may want to review the following with your parent to give him/her an opportunity to think through his/her choices and decisions before giving information to a lawyer.

1. Executor/executrix:
   a) Who are the most appropriate person(s) to serve as your executor or executrix?
   b) Who would you name if the above were no longer available?
2. To whom are you leaving your estate?
   a) all to one named beneficiary?
   b) divided equally between a number of named beneficiaries, i.e. family or friends
   c) proportioned into several bequests specific to a number of named beneficiaries, i.e. caregivers, housekeepers, doctors, etc.
   d) proportioned bequests to specific beneficiary institutions, charities, care homes, hospitals, etc.
3. Gifts to specific person(s) i.e. China set to a friend, car to a brother, or piece of jewellery to a sister, etc.
4. Alternative beneficiary(s) in case of a common disaster.
5. Two witnesses who are neither executor/executrix nor beneficiaries of your estate.

Step Two: Create an Appropriate Power of Attorney

Once the will is prepared ask your lawyer to also prepare a Power of Attorney (POA) document for each person to whom your parent is granting POA. Once these are signed and witnessed, make several copies – at least one for every regular service and legal/financial communication your parent receives. Have a few 'extras' in the file in case they are required from unexpected sources.

A Certified copy of the POA will be required by all financial/investment institutions, all sources of income i.e. annuities, pensions, and all government departments. You may find that one branch of government doesn't communicate with the others and each will require their own POA. You will also have to submit a POA to all organizations and services to which your parent subscribes. You may not be able to have telephone services or other utilities installed, moved or disconnected without such authority on file. It is best to systematically submit a POA everywhere relevant to simplify communications in future. It is important to note that power of attorney ends at the moment of death and responsibility is assumed by the executor(s).

Step Three: Move Assets Outside of the Will

Legally, a will requires a process called probate. Simply put, probate requires that the court certify that an individual or individuals have the right to administer the estate of a deceased person. The fees associated with this process vary from jurisdiction to jurisdiction. They may be assessed at a flat rate or at a percentage of the entire estate. Specific terms such as probate fees, death taxes, etc., will differ depending where the will is being probated.

The protection of one's assets, the reduction of stress and frustration often borne by executor(s), and avoidance of 'probate fees/taxes' and associated auxiliary costs, have become an integral part of estate planning.

There are two ways to remove assets from the will, each relevant to specific assets.

1. Assign a living beneficiary (not Estate) to all insurance policies, pensions, registered instruments, annuities, income funds, etc. This allows transfer of ownership to the beneficiary(s) without having to be processed through a will. Check each policy or contact your parent's insurance and financial agents to verify that a living beneficiary has been named.

2. Ensure all properties, vehicles, cash accounts and investments are held jointly with right of survivorship by one or more beneficiary or executor. The process to add your name to existing accounts is a relatively simple transaction between you, your parent and the banking, investment, or appropriate legal/government agencies.

- Transferring the title of property(s) to reflect joint ownership may require the services of a notary or lawyer. Contact the local government office responsible for land titles registry and ask for their guidelines and processes.

- The process of transferring ownership of a vehicle may vary from jurisdiction to jurisdiction. Contact the motor vehicle branch or your insurance agent to find out how to have your name (and/or that of another beneficiary) put on the ownership of the vehicle. It may be, your parent will have to sell you the car, relinquish the license plates and apply for a new license plate and subsequent insurance in both or just your name(s).

Apart from simplifying the disposition of assets after death, joint ownership allows you to conduct financial transactions on behalf of your parent should they be unable to do so themselves. There may come a time when even simple banking activities become impractical or even impossible.

Many of our parents own their own home, have more than one bank account and may deal with more than one financial institution. Some may also own or have interest in additional properties, have diversified investments and receive income from a variety of sources. How can you ensure that all assets have been identified and transferred to joint ownership or living beneficiary?

Step Four: Manage Asset Ownership

The first step in any change process is to create a base line. In this case, it is essential to create an inventory of all your parent's assets that require ownership on title or a beneficiary designation, listing pertinent details that will help manage and organize the transfer of ownership as well as simplify the process of disposition when the time comes. Do you know where all your Parent's assets are? Do you know which financial organizations they have dealt with over their lifetime? Could they have a 'secret account' long forgotten? Currently The Bank of Canada holds monies from unclaimed bank accounts. In the United States there is no central repository for unclaimed assets; these are managed on a state by state basis. Most of these assets can be traced online by going to the following Web sites:

http://www.bankofcanada.ca/unclaimed-balances/how-to-claim/

http://usgovinfo.about.com/od/moneymatters/a/ unclaimedstates.htm

The process for claiming such assets can be complicated. It's always best to ensure that all assets are listed and held jointly.

The Asset Inventory templates at the end of this section are provided to assist with this organization and to highlight specific assets that require either a living beneficiary or transfer to joint ownership with right of survival status. Look through these sheets, completing any section you can before collaborating with your parent. Forms can often be overwhelming and completed information can serve as an example, thereby simplifying the process as you discuss each point with your parent.

As you approach this project it may be prudent to first set goals, objectives and a reasonable time line for completing each task. This will help keep you on track as well as offer encouragement as you add a check mark to your to-do list. Seeing your progress in 'black and white' may help overcome the sense of being overwhelmed that could occur if the entire project is seen as one step. It is also important to avoid over taxing your parent's focus and/or energy.

Once you have completed the Property Asset Inventories© and identified which assets require change, see if there are several that can be dealt with at one time. Are there multiple properties, vehicles etc. that require transfer to joint ownership? Clumping like tasks together will simplify the process as well as save time, energy and even money if they require the services of a notary or lawyer.

Talk with your parent throughout the process, involving them at all stages. How would they like to proceed? Ensure your siblings and other potential beneficiaries are aware of what is happening. Discuss how this will simplify life for them and for the family. Make the entire process as positive and as open for your parent as possible.

Step Five: Inventory all General Assets

This fifth and final step in managing your Parent's assets often precedes the popular activity called downsizing. It is not the purpose of this exercise, however, to assume that your Parent is preparing to leave the family home. In fact, many seniors prefer to remain in their homes and address changes in abilities in a variety of ways detailed in the 'Supporting Independence'© section. Often, however, there comes a time when it is prudent for your parent to move into an environment where their needs and wants can be met in a safe and comfortable manner.

Whether an immediate move is pending or not, an inventory of specific assets can help your parent make informed decisions.

- Are there items s/he would want to keep no matter where s/he lives?
- Are there items s/he no longer want or need? Can these be sold, given away or donated to a worthy cause?
- Are there special items or collections that s/he would like to gift to a specific person? Would s/he prefer to do this before death or via a bequest?

There are many decisions to make, but first begin by creating an inventory of general household assets. As with the property assets, a series of 'General Asset Inventory'© forms are included to help simplify this process. You will notice each is divided into general categories: collections, sets, pairs, and general household items.

As you and your parent work through an inventory of his/her assets, you may identify items that can immediately be designated as items to sell, consign, donate to a charity, or recycle. Disposing of these items will help to clear space for your parent to truly appreciate the asset s/he has collected over the years as well as allow for the grouping of collections, etc., to better display total value when you have them appraised by a collectibles agent or antique expert.

The inventory asset sheets will help to organize this process. It is important to remember that this is a step-by-step process, designed to help your parent manage their assets and simplify their lives. Conducting this inventory will greatly assist both you and your parent should the time come to leave the family home.

As you begin your asset inventory, you may want to start with easy decisions. This is your parent's life, begun long before you were aware of the world around you. Collaborate with your parent, discuss their thoughts, opinions, wishes and share your own in a non-judgmental way. Remember to pace the process.

Enjoy the trips down memory lane as you share remembrances. Many items have their own story or figure prominently in fond memories of family life. This may be an emotional journey for both of you. Be kind to yourselves and allow the laughter and tears, knowing you are sharing a project that will help you both to simplify each other's lives – now and in the future.

Property Asset Inventory

LEGAL AND FINANCIAL MANAGEMENT
Property Asset Inventory©

Inventory - All Property Assets	$ Value	Location/ Address	Mortgage Holder or Co-Owner	Phone Number	Contact Name
Residences					
Clear					
Mortgaged					
Shared(Co-Owners)					
Additional Property (1)					
Clear					
Mortgaged					
Shared (Co-Owners)					
Additional Property (2)					
Clear					
Mortgaged					
Shared (Co-Owners)					

Additional Properties may include rental houses, apartment buildings, warehouses, storage yards, etc. These property assets all require joint ownership

Vehicular Asset Inventory

LEGAL AND FINANCIAL MANAGEMENT
Vehicular Asset Inventory©

Vehicle Assets	Vehicle Type	$ Value	Location/ Address	Motor Vehicle Branch - Phone Number	Insurance Agency - Contact Name	Insurance Agency - Phone Number
Vehicle (1)						
Owned						
Leased						
Loans						
Vehicle (2)						
Owned						
Leased						
Loans						
Vehicle (3)						
Owned						
Leased						
Loans						
Vehicle (4)						
Owned						
Leased						
Loans						
Vehicle (5)						
Owned						
Leased						
Loans						

All vehicular assets must be jointly owned. Vehicles include any machine licensed for public roads, e.g. Pick-up trucks, Motorcycles, trailers, 5th wheels, motor-homes.

Financial Asset Inventory (Cash)

LEGAL AND FINANCIAL MANAGEMENT
Financial Asset Inventory (Cash)©

Inventory - All Cash Assets	*Value*	Institution/ Location	Account Number(s)	Agent of Record	Phone Number
Cash Accounts					
Chequing					
Savings					
Term Deposits					
Guaranteed Investment Certificates (GIC)					
Treasury Bills					
Other					

Financial Asset Inventory (Investments)

LEGAL AND FINANCIAL MANAGEMENT
Financial Asset Inventory (Investments)©

Inventory - All Investment Assets	Value	Location	Account Number(s)	Agent of Record	Phone Number
Investments					
Stock Portfolio					
Bond Portfolio					
Mutual Funds					
Other					

All Non-Registered investments require Joint Ownership

Financial Asset Inventory (Pensions and Insurance)

LEGAL AND FINANCIAL MANAGEMENT
Financial Asset Inventory (Pensions and Insurance)©

Inventory - All Pension and Insurance Assets	Value	Location	Account Number(s)	Agent of Record	Phone Number
Government Registered Plans e.g. RRSP's, IRA's					
Pensions (OAP, CPP, Social Security, GIS, superannuation, military, disability, etc.)					
Registered Retirement Income Fund (RRIF) or Annuity					
Insurance - Life					
Insurance - Disability					

Pensions may include Old Age Security, Social Security, Canada Pension, career related pensions, spousal pensions,These plans all require a designated living beneficiary. Disability pensions, military pensions.

House and Garden Asset Inventory

LEGAL AND FINANCIAL MANAGEMENT
House and Garden Asset Inventory©

Asset	Value	Location	Details	Other Information

House and Garden Assets may include Furniture, Electronics, Dishes, Photographs, House Plants, Lawn Mowers, Snow Blowers, Gardening Tools, Power Tools, Hammers, etc.

Household Asset Inventory (Pairs, Sets, Collections)

LEGAL AND FINANCIAL MANAGEMENT
House and Garden Asset Inventory©
(Pairs, Sets and Collections)

Item	Number of Pieces	Description/Details	Location	Value

This Category may include coins, stamps, fine china, paintings, special plants (e.g. Orchids)

Disposition of Specific Gifts

LEGAL AND FINANCIAL MANAGEMENT
Disposition of Specific Gifts©

GIFT	DETAILS	RECIPIENT	DATE	
			NOW	BEQUEST
Example: Dish Set	Twelve Place Set: Spode India Tree	Grand-daughter Taylor	√	

Supporting an Independent Lifestyle

Life is short and we never have enough time for gladdening the hearts of those who travel the way with us. Oh, Be swift to love! Make haste to be kind.
Henri Frédéric Amiel

There are many subtle (and some not so subtle) ways of supporting and/or enhancing an independent lifestyle that help to meet the needs of all involved. If these enhancements can be promoted as 'making life easier' or 'freeing up time for more enjoyable activities', or simply 'too mundane to be bothered with anymore', it will be easier for your parent to accept. As with most things, it may be less intrusive to introduce change as a convenience rather than a 'cure' for what could be perceived as a failure or worse, the loss of abilities.

Before exploring some of the aids or options designed to supplement and compensate for physical, mental or emotional limitations, you need to examine ways to create and maintain a high degree of safety within and around your parent's home. If your parent lives in an apartment or condominium, the owner/manager of the building should assume responsibility for safety and maintenance of common interior areas as well as the exterior of all property.

If, however, your parent lives in a private home, it may be well worth your while and financial commitment, to have your parent's home inspected by a reputable contractor or company. Failing eyesight or loss of hearing acuity may not pick up potential dangers such as gas leaks, decaying decks or stairs, unsafe or overloaded wiring. Awkward, cramped or overcrowded spaces may lead to injuries and bunched or scattered rugs are an invitation to serious falls.

Apart from overloaded or worn wiring, the average home may have any number of potential fire hazards. Flammable substances should be kept well away from any heat source e.g. toasters, ovens, registers or baseboard heaters, boiling kettles or other cooking devices. Old newspapers, magazines and books should be sorted and either thrown out or donated appropriately. Oil, solvents, paint cans, and cleaning products should be kept in a well ventilated area and disposed of safely when past their expiry date or before, if no longer used.

Who would you call to conduct such an inspection? You may want to begin with your local fire department. If they don't conduct inspections themselves, they may know reputable organizations that will. Failing that, you may want to check with your county or municipal offices. Once a service visit is scheduled, it may be prudent to arrange for a family member or close neighbor to be present during the inspection. Finally, ask for a written report with recommendations.

A list of potential household/yard hazards is included at the end of this section together with a form for recording emergency and non-emergency service numbers. Creating a safe and secure environment within which your parent can enjoy a full and hazard-free lifestyle, is the first step in supporting their independence. The following section explores some options and services for augmenting an independent lifestyle by ensuring appropriate personal, medical, environmental, and emotional support is in place.

Support for Daily Living

Although your parent may appear to keep up with regular activities and social commitments, their body is aging and often with increasing limitation comes the need for increasing support.

Following are some of the more common 'aids' or service options that augment independence. In some cases, introducing these systems or products, before they are needed, eases the transition.

Medication Blister Packs

The changes inherent with aging often necessitate taking a variety of daily medications. Few argue about the need for a disciplined approach to taking the correct dosage at the prescribed time each day. However, there is significant concern around the negative impact age-related memory loss could have on a daily medication ritual. Seniors have been known to skip one or more doses and compensate by taking several at one time. To avoid confusion and possible health reactions to random doses, most pharmacists will package the necessary supplements and prescription drugs in a single blister pack. Pre-printed with times and days of the week, this is a simple way to organize and manage daily prescriptions or other medications rather than having to store and sort through an assortment of packages and bottles.

At the request of the family physician, or in some cases, the patient or representative, the pharmacist will arrange the correct dosage of daily medications, vitamins and/or pain relief on a segmented, plastic-covered card. At a glance, you can see which medications are taken at various times of day, generally at meals and bedtime.

It is also obvious if a dosage has been skipped. Your parent needs to know what to do if this occurs. Does s/he call the doctor/pharmacist, skip that dose, or double up (rarely is this recommended)? You may want to check out the used card(s) now and then to ensure that your parent understands the process and isn't skipping one or more sets of pills regularly. Blister Packs are generally prepared a week in advance and can be altered by the physician when necessary.

With a little bit of up front organization, patience, and diligence, your parent's medication routine will be simplified and contained. Use the following screening criteria to check out the pharmacies that deliver to your parent's neighborhood:

- Do they accept your parent's drug plan?
- Will they bill the drug plan directly?
- Will they send monthly statements for residual amounts or (better still),
- Will they charge additional costs to a credit card as they occur?
- Are their dispensing fees competitive?
- Do they offer discounts or other incentives to regular or senior customers?

69

- Do they have a set delivery schedule?
- Can a regular delivery time be scheduled to accommodate your parent's routine?
- Will they deliver non-prescription orders along with regular blister packs i.e. personal or grocery items? There may come a time when product delivery becomes necessary.

Remember to provide the details of your parent's health/drug plan(s) and, if appropriate, credit card information to the pharmacist and let your parent's physician know the contact information for the pharmacy you have chosen. The physician's office will work with the pharmacy to ensure all prescriptions/medications are current and packaged correctly.

If possible, it may be prudent to have the doctor and/or pharmacist explain and demonstrate how the Blister Pack system will simplify the process of ensuring that the right amount of medication is taken at the right time each day. At the same time, they can answer any questions your parent may have including:

1. What if I skip a pill one day?
   - Do I include with the next meal?
   - Do I double up the next day?

- Do I save and return to the pharmacist for a refund? (This has been known to happen.)

It is important that the responses to these questions are specific to each medication included in the blister pack and posted where your parent can review if necessary - could be stapled to a calendar or address book or even the original blister pack (which will be kept handy). You may also want to keep a copy of medications and when they should be taken. This list could be invaluable information for emergency medical or hospital personnel.

2. What if my delivery doesn't arrive when scheduled? Glitches happen. Be sure to schedule weekly delivery a day or so before the new blister pack is needed. This will allow your parent time to alert the pharmacy that the delivery didn't arrive on schedule BEFORE the current pack runs out.

3. What if my physician changes prescriptions, daily doses, or deletes/adds new prescriptions? You will want to have this discussion with both the physician and pharmacist to ensure that they are working as a team to ensure a smooth transition to changed medications.

In-Home Laboratory Services

The dosage of some medications is dependent on the results of regular laboratory tests. You may want to speak with your parent's physician about setting up a 'standing-order' for regularly scheduled in-home lab tests. If possible, schedule these appointments to fit into your parent's routine and request a phone call the day before or even the morning of the appointment to jog your parent's memory. As with all change, the smoother it is integrated into your parent's routine, the more likely it will be seen as an advantage rather than a threat to independence.

You will want to confirm that your parent's health plan(s) will cover this service without additional charges. If there are additional fees for this on-going service, see if you can arrange for surplus costs to be charged to a credit-card so you/your parent can minimize the number of monthly invoices and/or necessity for excessive cash in the home at any given time.

Medical Alert Systems

In-home accidents and medical emergencies are cause for considerable concern for seniors living alone. There are a number of services that will link your parent, via a necklace, bracelet, etc., to an emergency contact whose first responsibility is to check to see if help is needed or if the device was activated by mistake.

It may also be prudent to have an ID bracelet made for your parent listing an emergency contact number and any medical conditions. As well, you will want to ensure that your parent carries a card in their wallet with similar information as well as whom to call if disoriented and wandering away from home.

Some families have organized a rotation schedule that ensures that at least one member calls their parent every day or so. Apart from the social contact that so many seniors crave, the calls ensure that their parent is safe and well. If not, then assistance can be immediately forthcoming.

Telephone Shopping and Delivery

Many seniors enjoy shopping. Some make it a social event by joining friends as they move from one store to another, commenting on what each is buying and why. This is often the one area that folks resist giving up, in spite of increasing physical limitations.

Many local grocery stores offer telephone shopping and even free delivery over a certain amount; several offer professional pharmaceutical services as well. This may be a consideration when selecting your parent's pharmacy. There may come a time when having groceries delivered with the weekly blister pack significantly eases your parent's and your burden.

To simplify this process and avoid confusion over products with which your parent isn't familiar, you may want to go shopping with him/her to observe their decision making process.

What determines choices for your parent? Is it familiar brands or products? Is it the lowest price or a product on sale? Is it something they have wanted to try after seeing it advertised? Or, is it simply the desire to try something new?

Whatever influences your parent's choices, they are their choices and are not subject to judgment or debate; unless your advice is asked for, don't offer it. Of course, if there are health issues at stake, you will want to choose your words very carefully. If your parent has a condition that precludes excessive sugar, starch or fat, for example, you may have to direct their attention to products offering less. Your doctor can lend credibility to these choices as well. Don't hesitate to engage his/her help with issues pertaining to the health of your parent. If you have the opportunity, you may want to introduce the pharmacist to your parent. Putting a face to the service may help your parent accept changes or additions to his/her blister pack. It will also help to have professional health advice should your parent choose a product not suitable for existing conditions.

It may not be geographically possible for you or another family member to accompany your parent to the grocery store, however, the two of you can compile a master shopping list over time, leaving room for sale items and treats. You can contribute significantly to the list and to the success of the process by making a memory game out of it. Remembering all the foods you both enjoyed when you were young, will kindle fond memories of another time. Be sure to keep a current copy of this list as it will serve as a guide when your parent (or one day, you) place a call for groceries.

Again, it is prudent to check out the local stores, asking about discounts, delivery times and charges, billing arrangements, etc. Most of all, you want your parent to feel comfortable. The more familiar the products, the store, and the ordering process, the more likely your parent will continue it. The more comprehensive its services and products, the more effective telephone ordering/delivery will be in future. One stop shopping also eliminates running around to several stores.

Pre-Cooked/Frozen Meals

Some seniors welcome the chance to reduce the number of meals they need to prepare every week. Most grocery stores offer prepared dishes, fresh or frozen, which take little time to heat. Many of these are prepared to accommodate specific health requirements and are often as tasty as homemade. Some cities have stores that offer only frozen dishes, many in individual serving sizes. Check also with your parent's favorite grocery store for a list of food prepared and packaged in smaller sizes to accommodate a person living alone.

'Meals-On-Wheels' is a volunteer-based program offered in most cities and metropolitan areas of North America, the United Kingdom and Australia. Talk with your parent's physician to see if this service is available and appropriate for your parent. The program offers a variety of meal plans and menus from which your parent can select dishes in preferred quantities.

Fortunately, meals either arrive hot or can be easily frozen and reheated quickly for later use. There are selections prepared to accommodate specific dietary and often cultural requirements; all are nutritionally balanced, tasty and packaged in sizes appropriate to senior appetites.

The cost of this service depends on a variety of criteria but is generally related to the amount of food selected, and in some cases, the degree of financial need.

House/Yard Maintenance

Whether your parent lives in a house, condominium or apartment, there are cleaning and maintenance responsibilities inherent with living independently. There will be tasks your parent enjoys and is quite capable of performing, while others are less favored and seen as hard work. It is the latter you need to assess first.

Would your parent consider a private or commercial cleaning/maintenance service on a regular basis? Services can be as simple as a group of neighbors hiring a local teenager to dedicate an hour a week to each lawn or garden. Another option is for friends in the same apartment or condo to 'share' the services of a cleaning person scheduled to spend time in each home on the same day. Laundry services can be coordinated the same way, as most private apartments/condos have in-suite laundry facilities. The cost of these services will be less if shared by others as travel time and expenses are considerably less for the service provider.

CAUTION: *If your parent agrees to accept help with the more mundane tasks associated with living independently, it is best to formalize the arrangement by setting down specific tasks to be done as well as the schedule for service. A simple agreement will clarify types and frequencies of services provided, and hopefully, prevent inconsistency or cancellation by either party. An independent person may not want to be tied down to a specific schedule, seeing a chance to shop with friends more important than being home to admit a cleaning lady. S/he also might resent having to arrange their schedule to allow a stranger to do 'what I can do anyway'. Giving up tasks, even those we don't particularly enjoy may be viewed as a loss of control, and therefore something to avoid or sabotage.*

Organize and Simplify a Schedule

To simplify your parent's schedule and to assist with memory, have your parent schedule standing appointments whenever possible. Personal services such as hair, nails, podiatry services etc., can often be scheduled at the same time/day on a weekly, monthly or bi-monthly basis.

Create standing appointments for health-related services such as physiotherapy, massage therapy, chiropractic, dental and even medical. By including religious, social and community activities, your parent's calendar will quickly become very full. Creating established appointment times helps to sort activities into regular spots, leaving room for special events.

You may want to consider getting or updating a low-limit credit card in both your names against which all costs associated with your parent's daily living are charged. Depending on your relationship with the financial institution issuing the card, you may also wish to have the card paid from a specific account. This eliminates the need for your parent to keep excessive cash in their home or on their person. It also allows you to monitor expenditures and ensure that your parent's monthly medical, household, grocery, utilities, and personal grooming expenses are paid, even if you are out of town or unavailable to make such payments. The goal is not to take control away from your parent but to ensure s/he is able to maintain independence as long as physically, mentally and emotionally possible.

The Master Calendar

Once you and/or your parent have put some or all of these time and energy savers in place, you may want to create a Master Calendar noting the days/dates of regular appointments, deliveries, meetings, outings, services, etc. At the beginning of each month transfer this information into a calendar or date book. Once these new processes have integrated themselves into your parent's routine, you may want to consider preparing a master calendar of all standing appointments and having a few printed for those family members close to your parent. If you choose, you may even put your parents' schedule on an electronic calendar such as Google or Yahoo, and give all family members access. This will allow everyone to connect their personal mobile device to the Calendar and receive notifications and alerts whenever a significant event or activity is scheduled. That way, regular social calls from family members can also be 'soft' reminders of the day's activities. It also shows your parent others are interested in her/his routine and habits. Support comes in many forms. Some folks value their privacy; others enjoy sharing the daily activities with family and friends. You will know which works best for your parent; if not initially, then certainly after a period of trial and error. Parents have a way, subtle or not, of letting you know when you over-step their boundaries. Ah, if only that awareness could work as well the other way.

It may be wise to encourage your parent to establish regular outings with friends for those days free of other commitments. If given a choice of waiting for the lab technician or cleaning person, or going out with friends, few would stay at home.

A Final Thought

Helping your parent maintain their independence may seem time consuming and indeed there will be considerable up-front activity to ensure the smooth integration of the support 'aids' discussed to this point. However, it pales beside the amount of time, worry, energy and frustration you could devote to rectifying missed appointments, mismanaged or skipped medications and decline in personal and environmental hygiene. At the end of the section, you will find a number of information sheets and/or guides to help you decide which of these aids best suit your parent's lifestyle at this point. You will want to review this chapter as your parent's abilities and skills evolve. As with all change, if you are able to create the impression (real or illusion) that these changes are the will of your parent, whatever initiative you integrate, will have a much better chance of success.

Regular Appointment Schedule

SUPPORTING INDEPENDENCE
Regular Appointment Schedule

Support Services	Contact Name	Contact Number	Standing App'ts Y or N	Date & Time	Costs	Notes
Personal Care						
Hair						
Manicure						
Pedicure						
Other						
Social						
Spiritual						
Community						
Other						
Recreation						
Fitness						
Sports						
Community						
Other						

Regular Bill Payments

SUPPORTING INDEPENDENCE
Regular Bill Payments

Support Services	Contact Name	Contact Number	Standing Appt's. Y or N	Date & Time	Costs	Notes
Medical						
Physician						
Physician Specialists						
General Health						
Chiropractor						
Dentist						
Laboratory						
Massage Therapist						
Naturopath						
Optometrist						
Physio-therapist						
Audiologist						
Health Insurance						
Extended Health Insurance						

SUPPORTING INDEPENDENCE
Regular Bill Payments

Creditor	Name	Address	Phone	Amount Due	Payment Date*	Notes
Financial						
Mortgage/Rent						
Associated Fees						
Debt Servicing						
Insurance						
House						
Automobile						
Life						
Disability						

*How many of these can be automatically paid through the financial institution to eliminate the need for monthly checks to be mailed and processed? See Legal and Financial Section for details.

SUPPORTING INDEPENDENCE
Regular Bill Payments

Creditor	Name	Address	Phone	Amount Due	Payment Date	Notes
Utilities						
Maintenance						
Cleaning						
Telephone						
Internet						
Cable						
Electric						
Heat						
Water						
Pharmacy						
Newspaper						
Memberships						
Other						

*How many of these can be automatically paid through the financial institution to eliminate the need for monthly checks to be mailed and processed? See Legal and Financial Section for details.

Potential Hazard Check Sheet (House and Yard)

SUPPORTING INDEPENDENCE
Potential Hazard Check Sheet© - In Home

Hazard	Risk	Solution	Notes
Rugs	Tripping	Removal	
Gas Stoves	Fire		
	Asphyxiation	Switch to Electric	
Bathrooms	Slipping & Falling	Rails	
	Inaccessibility	Shower Stalls	
Medications	Over/Under dose	Blister Packs	
Stairs	Falling	Dual Hand Rails	
		Good Stair Treads	
Wiring	Fire	Replace Faulty Wiring	
Extension Cords	Tripping	Complete Removal, Relocation	
Portable Heaters	Fire & Tripping	Complete Removal	
Storage	Inaccessibility	Avoid High/Low placement	
	Standing on Chairs/Step-Stools		

SUPPORTING INDEPENDENCE
Potential Hazard Check Sheet© - Garden

Hazard	Risk	Solution	Notes
Garden Tools	Heart and Circulatory Stress	Restrict heavy lifting, digging, or throwing	
		Use only light duty gear such as trowels	
Power Tools	Cuts, Punctures, Burns	Restrict usage to times when younger family members present	
Ladders	Falling	Restrict Usage	
Other			

Role Clarification

...this above all, to thine own self be true...
Hamlet (Act I, Scene 3) William Shakespeare

Wanting to live independently and being independent are very different concepts. It is important for you to determine your role as you begin the process of putting support aids in place for your parent. It could be very easy for you to slip into the role of primary caregiver, housekeeper, best friend and/or general servant.

What are your expectations of your role? Perhaps even more important, what are your parent's expectations of your role? You may want to revisit the Family of Origin Responsibility Chart© you completed at the end of the *Perceptions and Expectations* Section. Think about your parent's role(s) as you were growing up. Did s/he assume responsibility for themselves, for the family, for an extended family, or was your parent content to abdicate control to others? How did your parent view his/her responsibility to you and/or your siblings? Were you seen as dependents needing care or as support to ease your parent's physical or emotional burdens? Take a good look at the kinds of relationships your parent forms. Are they mutually supportive? How does your parent perceive the role of his/her friends? As your parent has aged, are friends seen as comrades, sharing the joys of conversation and social activities? Or, are they viewed as folks who will take care of and be there for, your parent?

The parent who wants to maintain control of his/her daily routine, may also hesitate to allow strangers into their realm, preferring to have family or friends perform supportive services. The self-focused parent sees only their needs and will think nothing of burdening a friend, neighbor or adult child with unreasonable or inappropriate responsibility. There are parents who feel it is their children's duty to care for them as they age. They see themselves as the only priority and have spent a significant part of their lives honing the art of manipulation by guilt. Remember your parent(s) made their choices throughout their life. Their attitudes, mental health and to a large degree, their physical condition, are the results of those choices.

Loss of control can be very frightening to someone who is beginning to slow down. Folks tend to fall back on old habits during times of stress or pressure. If your parent's habit was to hide or camouflage illness or unpleasantness, you need to be alert for subtle signs of increasing limitations. Take a moment to review the Record of Change© document at the end of *This Thing Called Independence* section. What kind of behavioral changes will alert you to increased limitations and the potential need for external resources?

If, alternatively, your parent's habit has been to transfer difficulty to you or others, the demand for attention and assistance may significantly increase. It is best to have researched, selected and implemented appropriate external resources before a crisis situation (real or imagined) draws you into a role you are not able or willing to fulfil on a long-term basis. The degree to which external resources need to be integrated depends on the nature and extent of the gaps they are intended to bridge. Completion of the Role Clarification Chart© at the end of this section will enable you to identify various gaps in care and manage this process efficiently and effectively.

At some point, many sense that the parent-child role is reversing. While this can be a natural progression, it is important to be aware that it is happening. Know your own limitations, what you are able to do and give. Going beyond this point can cause excessive worry, frustration and even exhaustion. Your parent is your parent. You have known them all your life. You have an image of them that may be swaddled in childhood fantasy or shrouded by teenage anxiety and frustration.

Seek to know your own, and your parent's, sense of reality. Who and what is your parent now? What are their dreams, their goals, and their wishes? What matters to them? How far will they go to achieve their objectives? Finally, if at all possible, discover what their expectations are for, and of, you.

Does your parent wish you a life of peace and happiness, free of the pressures inherent in growing a family and/or career? Do they view you as an independent, successful person living life as you choose? Or, do they see you as their support and themselves as your priority?

Along with your perceptions and understanding, it is your responsibility to frame the current relationship with your parent. How do you see it unfolding; as it always has? Does this work for you? If not, what can or will you do to subtly change this?

Change can take people out of their comfort level, causing anxiety and often anger. You might want to spend some time observing rather than responding to the interactions that don't work for you. Is there something that you could have done before or immediately after things went 'off the rails'? Or is it simply that you compromise what is best for you rather than refuse or deny your parent? If so, it is up to you to determine what works for you and your parent and devise ways to ensure a healthy balance.

Are you willing to fill the role of spouse or best friend, of devil's advocate or decision maker, of primary caregiver or domestic help? How does being a daughter or son fit into your parent's and your own perceptions?

Take the time to define your role and how best to integrate it incrementally into your interactions with your parent. The Role Clarification© chart included with this section is designed as a guide to help you with this process. It is a given that every person and therefore every situation, is unique. Your relationship with an aging parent cannot be patterned after anyone else's. If you have the privilege of discussing their evolving situation with your parent, try to raise any concerns or questions regarding your relationship now and in future.

Remember, if your parent is looking for a servant, it is not you. Find ways of changing patterns when you begin to absorb more and more of your parent's daily maintenance and social needs, while they insist on making independent choices and decisions. Avoid being the safety net for rash or foolish actions taken simply to assert independence or for spite.

Your role is to work with your parent (if possible) to alleviate the physical, emotional and social burdens on them, without placing yourself in the position of picking up the slack.

Defining your role and that of your parent can take on many forms. For instance, in consultation with your parent, you may agree to research and arrange payment for yard work, house cleaning, laundry, grocery delivery, etc. In return, your parent agrees to accept and give access to these services at agreed upon times. It is essential that your parent understand that this isn't just a casual chat but an arrangement that will govern specific aspects of your interactions.

It may be necessary for you to draw up individual 'contracts' between your parent and external resources outlining the specific role(s) and responsibilities of each party. Sample agreements are included at the end of this section. If possible, have a trusted friend of your parent or other respected family member formally witness such agreements. This may help to avoid the temptation to change or cancel arrangements just to spite you or to prove s/he is capable of managing their own affairs without your interference. The motivation behind such an action could be the desire to have you perform the tasks yourself. If you suspect this is so, it would be prudent to consider what would lead to such reasoning and how best to modify such desires and/or transfer such responsibility to external resources.

Does this seem harsh, too formal, even bureaucratic? It may be that you are very comfortable with your relationship with your parent and therefore defining your role may not seem necessary. Again, take the time to think about your upbringing. Who held the family together? How were family members viewed? Is your parent a widow/widower? How has the loss of a spouse or partner impacted the way your parent interacts with friends and family today? Think through the overt or unspoken expectations your parent has of you. Are these okay? Are you willing for these expectations to increase as your parent continues to age? Clarifying and integrating your role is essential if you are to enjoy a mutually healthy and loving relationship with your parent. Again, the Role Clarification Chart© should help you begin this process.

Role Clarification Chart

ROLE CLARIFICATION CHART©

Activity	Self	Family (Name)	External Resources
		Contact Information	Contact Information
House Work			
Laundry			
Meal Preparation			
Clean-up			
Finance			
Banking			
Investments			
Bill Payments			
Shopping			
Personal Care			
Bathing			
Dressing			
Hair			
Nails			
Morning Routine			
Evening Routine			
Bed Time Routine			

ROLE CLARIFICATION CHART©

Activity	Self	Family Member (Name)	External Resources
Appointments			
Medical			
Transportation			
Emergency Help			
Other			

Sample Agreement (The Caregiver's Role)

1. Monitor prescription drugs

2. Assist with shower - assist with dressing as needed

3. Assist with and monitor personal hygiene

4. Apply topical medication when/where necessary

5. Weekly laundry of outer and inner wear - wash, dry, iron if necessary and put away

6. Sort, wash and pack away seasonal clothing on request

7. Light housekeeping: dishes, dusting, plant maintenance, disinfecting wipes, make bed, change if necessary, assist with sorting projects on request

8. Monthly cleaning of dishes using dishwasher

9. In consultation with client write weekly grocery list - shop for groceries on request

10. Accompany on appointments when necessary and requested

11. Accompany on walks if requested

12. Prepare and serve light meal, if requested

Signatures

Parent's Name _____

Your Name _____

Caregiver's Name _____

Witness _____

Sample Agreement (Client's Role)

1. Be open and communicate with Caregiver -let her know what is working for you, what isn't, why

2. Be patient if Caregiver does something different from your way talk about it openly

3. Always be home and ready to open the door when Caregiver arrives

4. Let family member know what is working, what you'd like to change and why

5. Use the time with your Caregiver wisely. She's the reason you can maintain your independence

6. Enjoy getting to know your Caregiver. Think of fun things you can do together

7. Take your medication every morning:Take the green pill at dinner and another at bedtime

8. Work with your caregiver to understand and maintain personal hygiene

9. Keep weekly hair appointments - to feel clean and well groomed

10. Jot down shopping needs on pad on microwave. Your caregiver/family member will use this list to ensure you never run out of anything

11. Put soiled pyjamas, underwear, and outer wear in laundry basket in storage cupboard. Your caregiver will wash everything weekly

12. Pile bank statements, bills, etc., on your dresser for family member's attention. You do not need to pay bills, respond to mail or fill out surveys.

Signatures

Parent's Name_____

Your Name _____

When Independence is Not Enough

Resolve to be tender with the young, compassionate with the aged, sympathetic with the striving, and tolerant with the weak and the wrong. Sometime in life you will have been all of these.

Bob Goddard

In the section entitled *This Thing Called Independence*, you completed the Record of Change Information Sheet© to help you and your parent understand when a change in behavior indicates that additional support is needed to complement an independent lifestyle.

There will come a time, however, when depending upon external resources may not be enough. A more consistent and continuous support of daily routine is required. Depending on available financial resources, there are a number of options to consider.

Let's look at the most traditional first. Historically, when a parent dies and the spouse is no longer able to cope on their own, s/he is invited to live with one or more of his/her adult children. Books, plays and even jokes have recorded both hilarious and tragic accounts of what happens within an existing family when Mom or Dad comes to live.

In the novel, The Stone Angel, Margaret Lawrence captures both the pain and frustration as an aging mother reluctantly relinquishes her independence, all the while stirring within the reader an understanding of, and empathy for, the much maligned daughter-in-law. It is a thought-provoking read that presents a very real picture of the challenges that can arise when an independent woman can no longer live on her own.

Does it have to be this way? No! In fact, some cultures are based on the care and reverence of elder relatives. It is expected that the nuclear family will expand to admit those unable to care for themselves. Children grow up knowing that one day their parent(s) will need to live with them, just as their grandparent(s) are an integral part of their daily routine.

Pioneer television captured the symbiotic relationship that developed when 'Gramps' moved in to replace an absent father and husband in the early episodes of Lassie.

In other cultures, it is the single adult child or newly married family that moves in with Mom and Dad, creating an environment conducive to mutual care and attention.

As societies have evolved, so too have traditional customs. While the respect and reverence of the elderly remains a priority today, some cultures have established retirement communities and care facilities unique to their own traditions, race or belief system.

Retirement and full care facilities may be sponsored and maintained by community service groups such as Rotary International, The Lions Club, Kinsmen, Knights of Columbus, and veteran support organizations, etc. In some cases, affiliation with a specific group is mandatory, but not always.

Most communities offer various levels of retirement and care facilities. Some of these may be privately owned and operate with fixed rates for specific accommodation and services. Others, publicly funded, may offer income-based subsidies for established care.

Local health authorities and/or service organizations often publish a grid listing the various kinds of senior accommodation and levels of care offered within the community. This and other information may be available on-line, in the telephone directory, or through a family doctor. As you work your way through the various options, you will want to record pertinent details and contact information for future reference. You will find a form to help with this process at the end of this section.

Before moving into an examination of what each level of care might entail, pause and consider what would work best in your own situation. What are your cultural norms? Would your parent be more comfortable living in an environment specific to his/her beliefs and traditions? What was your parent's home environment like? What kind of facility would best suit their taste and expectations? How active is your parent? What kinds of physical, mental, spiritual and social activities do they enjoy?

These are questions best broached as early in this process as possible. Have ongoing discussions with your parent, your siblings, and friends whose aging parents are facing similar decisions. Do your homework. Know what resources are readily available in your community and what the process is to access them. Use the Record of Change Information Sheet© as a gentle reminder to both you and your parent to revisit next steps and various contingencies as more assistance is required.

One way to encourage ongoing discussion of various residential options, is to walk or drive around your parent's (or your) neighborhood looking at various retirement/care homes. Although an appointment is generally needed for a comprehensive tour, you can tell a lot by walking through the front door of a facility. You might want to walk around the grounds, if accessible, first to give your parent a flavor of what others would see when visiting. How you are greeted and the information you receive will help 'flesh' out your first impression of the facility. Few of us would rent or buy a home without visiting it a few times. If would be unfair to have your parent move into a new home s/he has never even seen before.

Accommodation Options

The various levels of care provide a spectrum of services and activities. Some of these may be very important to your parent, some they would never use. It is best to know before you begin your search for appropriate accommodation what kinds of services and activities will contribute to your parent's successful integration into, and ongoing comfort with, a new environment. As well, there are facilities designed to include all levels of care, allowing a retirement living resident to evolve to assisted-living and eventually to full care services. Aging-in-place helps to avoid potential anxiety and confusion should it become necessary to increase the level of care.

As you work through this process, it is important to determine which services and activities are included in the monthly fee and which require additional payment. For instance, many facilities operate a small bus to regularly transport residents to shopping, financial and/or medical facilities. Some charge a fee for this service; others simply include such expenses in the monthly rate.

Some facilities offer medical alert systems that are attached to an on-site 24 hour reception/security area and are included in the cost of rent. Others do not offer 24 hour front desk services so medical alert services are maintained externally at the user's expense.

Arts and crafts, exercise classes, and in-house concerts or plays are often included in a monthly fee. However, special event meals, entertainment trips and personal services such as hair, nails, podiatrist etc., are usually out-sourced and financially supported by the users.

Some facilities offer a 'trust' program whereby an amount of money (over and above rental fees) is deposited into an internal 'trust' account for each resident. Activity fees, 'tuck' shop purchases as well as personal service expenses may be charged against this account. This allows residents to have control over minor purchases and grooming choices. It also provides a record that enables the external caregiver to keep track of how the 'trust' money is spent. Usually, when the resident is admitted, the external caregiver is given a choice of available services that can be accessed through the 'trust' fund. As your parent's needs change and/or the capacity for decision making diminishes, services can be added or deleted from daily, weekly or monthly routines.

The Personal Care and Physical Activity Base Line Chart© A & B, found at the end of this section, is designed to help you and your parent(s) identify the kinds of activities or services specific to your current and potential future needs. When completing this chart, remember what you are attempting to do is ensure continuity of service before, during, and after a change of accommodation. If a monthly nurse visit is part of your parents current support routine, will it be necessary for you to arrange this in the future, or will the new accommodation include this with the monthly fees? Similarly, if your parent has been doing their own laundry within their own home, will you wish to have self-serve laundry facilities available, or will you make a decision to switch to full laundry service?

Most facilities, private or publicly funded, offer a brochure, website, or a less formal information source that lists activities and services included in accommodation fees, as well as optional services that may be purchased either through the facility or privately.

While some facilities rent or offer space to accommodate on-site services such as hair salons or massage therapy facilities, others coordinate monthly appointments with external providers such as podiatrists, audiologists, etc., who will meet with residents in their own rooms. Fees for these services are generally handled directly by the resident.

Another consideration is appropriate storage and/or parking for motorized transport. Does the facility provide secure parking that is protected from the elements and allows access directly into the building?

Driving may not always be an option. Are there safe, attractive places for your parent to walk or sit outside? What about the immediate neighborhood? If your parent is fond of shopping, are there stores and services within walking distance? Could they walk to their bank, hairdresser, or grocery store? Is this important to them? If so, add it to their list of 'must haves'.

Apart from the level of care required and the resources available, it is important to understand how your parent wants to live. Is the desire for private accommodation the top priority? Not always. Some folks are not comfortable living on their own, especially if the move is prompted by the recent death of a spouse or partner. In this case, a dorm or ward situation might be acceptable, perhaps even preferred. Others, accustomed to managing their own space, would feel very confined sharing personal living quarters.

Personal accommodation within a facility can vary from a shared room; single bed, cupboard, end table, shared bathroom, to a private small room; single bed, end table, chair, dresser, cupboard, powder room, to large, multi-room apartments, complete with mini-kitchen (microwave, cupboards, sink, and fridge) and balcony. Again, it is prudent to not only know your parent's current needs and wants, but what kinds of considerations s/he may require in future. For instance, is the bathroom equipped with a raised toilet, a walk-in shower, accessible cupboards, sufficient counter space, and handrails?

In some States and Provinces, there are facilities that accommodate the transition from independent retiree to full care services. The concept of transitional living greatly interests some, while others are content to choose their accommodation one step at a time. It is not easy to imagine yourself totally dependent on others and unable to make even the simplest decisions.

The options are out there. As you work through the sheets at the end of this section, you and your parent will form a picture of how you each visualize the where, how and when of home.

REMEMBER: *When everyone leaves, it is your parent who will turn out his/her light at the end of the day. It is essential that their wishes be considered if at all possible. It is to everyone's advantage to ensure your parent is comfortable and feels at home.*

Private Facility Attributes

PRIVATE FACILITY ATTRIBUTES

Facility Name, Address and Telephone	Medic Alert	24 hr. Reception	House Keeping	Laundry	Phone	Cable	Parking	Kitchen	Bus	Meals	Personal Care	Common Space	Music Program	Exercise Equipment	Pool	Scheduled Activities	Elevator

F – Free

$ - Nominal Fee

Check all that Apply

Public Facility Attributes

PUBLIC FACILITY ATTRIBUTES

Facility Name, Address and Telephone	Medic Alert	24 hr. Reception	House Keeping	Laundry	Phone	Cable	Parking	Kitchen	Bus	Meals	Personal Care	Common space	Music Program	Exercise Equipment	Pool	Scheduled Activities	Elevator

F – Free

$ - Nominal Fee

Check all that Apply

114

Personal Care and Physical Activity Baseline Chart A

PERSONAL CARE and PHYSICAL ACTIVITY BASELINE CHART – A
Foundation Activities

Activity	Current	Future	Notes
Health Care			
Nurse Visit			
Lab Visit			
Audiology			
Other			
Personal Care			
Hair Salon			
Bathing			
Pedicure			
Manicure			
Other			
House-Keeping			
Linen/Laundry			
Personal Laundry			
Weekly 'Light' Cleaning			
Garbage Removal			
Other			

Personal Care and Physical Activity Baseline Chart B

PERSONAL CARE and PHYSICAL ACTIVITY
BASELINE CHART – B
Foundation Activities (continued)

Activity	Current	Future	Notes
Social			
Group Outings			
Group Activities			
Get Togethers 'In-House'			
Get Togethers Outside			
Recreation			
Cards			
Crafts			
Games			
Puzzles			
Library			
Other			
Food Preparation			
Shopping			
Cooking for Self			
Pre-Cooked Meals			
Guests for Meals			

Maintaining Mobility

We don't stop playing because we grow old. We grow old because we stop playing.

George Bernard Shaw

A major concern of the aging, and those who care for them, is the issue of mobility. As the population ages, the number of products and services that support, increase, or supplement mobility, is growing rapidly. Magazine features, television commercials, and advertisements posted on the walls of medical clinics, laboratories and health-related agencies, portray happy seniors taking advantage of the many support aids available to the public. While some of these aids may be appropriate for your parent now, many may not be needed for several years, if ever. Before exploring some of these options in detail, it is essential to emphasize the importance of your parent keeping active and fit, physically, mentally and emotionally.

How active is your parent? Is s/he involved socially? Is s/he engaged in regular group or individual exercise or do they depend on driving rather than walking even short distances. Do they still read their favorite authors or magazines? How often does your parent maintain relationships or interact with old friends? Is s/he open to meeting new acquaintances?

Milestone birthdays or the increasing aches and occasional pains of advancing years are not, in themselves, reasons for the self-imposed 'slowing down' that some seniors believe is natural. Unless there are physical limitations due to illness or accident, most seniors should be encouraged to maintain their regular routines, rituals, and relaxation patterns. They may wish to modify the duration, exertion level and even the frequency of their daily activities as required. However, knowing that they are still capable of enjoying life as they have chosen to live it is one of the best reinforcements for continued healthy living.

Physical Stamina and Flexibility

Discuss your parent's daily routine with them, focusing on any regular physical activity. Are there some adjustments needed to enhance safety and protection from injury or accident while encouraging ongoing flexibility? Inserting simple questions into regular chats may eliminate the fear of judgment or worry.

Similar to the Record of Change© document found elsewhere in this book, it is important for you and your parent to create an activity baseline detailing his/her activity levels at this point. How else can you measure changes when they occur? The Record of Physical Activity© chart at the end of this section is designed to help you and your parent identify and describe current activities. Together you may want to set reasonable goals or fitness targets. You may also want to use the chart as a springboard to discussions of how and when physical limitations can be accommodated. For example, the chart lists Walking/Running as a physical activity; however, this may be undertaken either individually or a group, so you would simply check the preferred choice. For this kind of activity the appropriate support would be high quality walking or running shoes, and you would write this under Support Required. Alternatively, if the person is only interested in horseshoes, then support may involve finding a location where horseshoes are played, as this can only be a group activity. Remember, it isn't necessary to complete every line in this chart; the most important consideration is to support and encourage your parent to continue those tasks, activities and events that make them happy and bring them joy.

There are some very basic adjustments to your parent's routine that will support and may even enhance their lifestyle. Perhaps the simplest yet often overlooked are attractive, functional and supportive shoes. Gone are the days when heavy, awkward, unattractive footwear were the only alternative to soft sided slip-on flats, strappy sandals, or designer pumps. Even the manufacturers of solid athletic, running shoes offer lines of attractively trim, leather shoes that provide support specific to the wearer's needs. These are easy to maintain, repair and some even come with a subtle zipper or Velcro that eliminates the challenge, and for the arthritic, the pain, of having to tie laces.

An attractive yet supportive shoe should be worn regularly, not kept just for outdoor activity or around the house. It will provide walking stability on rough or unpaved surfaces and help to offset tendencies to pronate or walk with an uneven gait. It will also prevent stumbles or falls caused by loose, low support shoes or slippers.

Structured Exercise

Apart from walking either for pleasure or as a means of transportation, there are many recreation organizations and senior centers that offer regular classes to promote and support well being, muscle strength, and flexibility. Some of the 'gentle' martial arts such as Tai Chi and She Ba Fah allow a gradual and relaxed process of incremental learning and similar to the many variations of Yoga, also enhance balance and relaxation.

If your parent prefers a more social activity, there are classes offered in dance; clog, square, polka being some of the more physical ones. For those who prefer a gentle yet beneficial routine, aqua fit or even regular swimming will meet their needs.

For those who prefer to exercise in private, there are a variety of home exercise machines designed to strengthen legs, arms and cardio-vascular systems. As well, there are plenty of interactive audio/video recordings that encourage fitness at specific levels. You may want to check your local library or senior center for appropriate resources before purchasing your own. Local television stations often offer fitness or strength building programs as well.

Along with a structured exercise program, it may be prudent to encourage massage, chiropractic or active release therapies to promote overall health.

If these activities or services are not familiar to your parent, don't push it. 'Soft' suggestion is often more effective than promoting something as the only way to go. Listen to what s/he is saying and the emotion(s) behind their words. Encourage

121

your parent to listen to their own bodies and adjust their activity and movement accordingly. Do their aches and pains reflect the lack of exercise or over exertion? Avoiding the use of sore muscles will not strengthen them. Failing to move joints regularly may cause them to stiffen. On the other hand, pushing far beyond comfort and safety may lead to accidents or injury, significantly compromising movement in future. It is important that your parent NOT over-compensate in either direction. A slow and steady adjustment from a sedentary lifestyle eliminates the soreness of overtaxed muscles while encouraging increased flexibility and energy.

Together, find what works best for them, what feels right. Encourage the integration into their daily and/or weekly routines until it becomes a habit, something done every day, like cleaning their teeth. 'If this is Tuesday, it must be Tai Chi' is a healthier approach than 'if this is Tuesday, my favorite show is on'. An established routine is a good reminder and a guide to effective time management as well as memory management. If your parent is aware of, and takes care of their body first, they will ultimately enjoy their favorite show for many more years. Nowhere is the adage 'use it or lose it' more evident than in the aging population.

Mobility Aids

There comes a time when the limitations of age begin to exert themselves with more than a passing twinge when we move position or realize the need to grasp the handrail when walking downstairs. The fear of falling becomes a reality as we sense our balance and stability becoming compromised. There are a number of aids to counter and/or support the impact of the march of time. Each one has its advantages and for some, its disadvantages. Let's take a look at some of the more popular options, knowing that this list is far from complete.

The Walking Cane

They come in many different designs, from the basic curved handle to the very ornately decorated handle; however, the most important thing to remember is that a cane must be measured to fit an individual. A cane that is too short encourages bending over and compromises the user's breathing and posture. In a worst case scenario, a short cane can be held responsible for rounded shoulders and a hump. If osteoporosis is a concern, then it is imperative that good posture be encouraged. A cane that is too long will not be held by the handle and becomes little more than a walking stick, compromising balance and stability, if it is carried at all.

The Walker

If your parent indicates an interest in a walker, there are several types to consider. But first, see how they do with grocery carts when they go shopping. If they are happy to relinquish your arm and whirl up and down the aisles, using the cart for the support and the balance they need, then they are ready for a walker.

At one end of the spectrum, there's the frame that precedes you as you walk. It is simply lifted and moved forward. Lacking wheels, it depends on the user for propulsion. At the other end of the scale, is a four wheel walker, complete with basket and a seat. The wheels can be locked and hand controls manage the brakes. It gives the sense of total freedom but has a seat in case a short rest is needed along the way. It is built to withstand and fit sidewalks, roads and uneven surfaces, as well as hardwood, tile and carpeted floors.

Similar to canes, walkers must be adjusted to the proper height for the user. While a simple adjustment, it may be necessary to adjust and re-adjust depending on an individual's need. Remember, this is a transition from leaning on an arm for support to forging ahead independently. It

124

is important that the height of the walker encourage the best possible posture; one that opens the airways and allows breathing to be a more natural and smooth process. By encouraging your parent to stand as straight as possible, you are helping them prevent rounded shoulders and a crooked spine, as well as potential respiratory compromise.

The Wheel Chair

Unless there is significant limitation, you may want to put off choosing a wheel chair in favor of encouraging the use of a cane or walker. Once the decision is made to move into a chair, it is seldom reversed. As with the other mobility aids, it is important to know beforehand what kind of wheel chair you are seeking. Models run the spectrum from the basic chair on wheels self- propelled by feet, right up to a motorized unit complete with tray and other attachments. There are as many considerations as there are options. You and your parent may want to research the system most appropriate for him/her before approaching a salesperson. Knowing what is needed ahead of time can avoid buying a system that is too simplistic or too complicated for their needs.

Perhaps the most significant concern is who is available to push the chair. Is it a means of transport to and from a dining room situation or will

125

it be used constantly even during the short ride to the bathroom. If your parent is living independently, then an independent chair, i.e. motorized, may be for him/her. If, however, they are generally assigned to nursing staff or to an aid, then it may be prudent to discuss this with their caregiver.

In any event, ensure that any decisions made reflect what your parent wants at this stage; once in a wheel chair, your parent may become increasingly dependent upon the chair and the caregiver.

These are the three major kinds of mobility aids; if you wish to try them, often the local Red Cross will lend or rent them for a specific period of time. Or, if you wish, you can buy them outright. In many cities, there are medical suppliers that will sell you 'gently' used equipment and take them back on consignment when you no longer need them.

Some of these additional aids are: raised toilet seats and bars to assist with lifting, shower/bath bars, and bed rails to help support and steady movement from one position to another. If balance and stability are issues, decorative hand bars may be placed throughout an apartment or house to ensure safety. You may want to walk through your parent's home and determine what, if anything is needed to increase their comfort and safety.

Transportation

Along with their personal mobility, it is essential to ensure the safety and security of your parent and others. One of the most precious symbols of independence is the possession of a valid driver's license. Most jurisdictions require that drivers over the age of 80 years take an annual driving test to ensure they are still alert enough to drive safely. The responsibility for ensuring the safety of the driver as well as the safety of others does not rest entirely on the licensing agency. It is a responsibility shared by the aging driver and by his/her family as well. Talk to your parent about driving before competence and/or safety become an issue.

A good number of potential problems could be solved by enrolling in a refresher driver training course designed specifically for seniors. Driving practices or attitudes that compromise or violate safety standards can be identified and worked on during subsequent lessons and practice sessions. Retraining may not work for all seniors, however a few areas that result in failure can be worked on before (and after) taking a test. These are:

- failure or inability to shoulder check (a good reason to continue to work on flexibility)
- failure to come to a complete stop at stop signs

127

- failure to turn into the correct lane.

It is far easier to correct bad habits and incomplete knowledge before an examination than to regain a driver's license after losing it. Check with your parent's insurance company or family doctor to see if counselling or driver refresher services are offered locally. Many jurisdictions have developed medical-fitness driver guidelines which define for physicians the adverse impact of specific medical conditions on driving.

You may wish to alert your parent's physician in advance of the potential need to administer a cognitive impairment test if you suspect that your parent's driving ability may be declining. For instance, The SIMARD MD is a valid and reliable screening tool for identifying cognitively impaired drivers whose driving skills may have declined to an unsafe level.[1]

'SIMARD MD' is an acronym for '**S**creen for the **I**dentification of Cognitively Impaired **M**edically **A**t-**R**isk **D**rivers a **M**odification of the **D**emTect'. It is called a modification of the DemTect (MD)[2] because it uses a subset of the items from that screening tool.

During casual conversations, encourage your parent to view their physician as part of his/her wellness team and let them know it's all right to share concerns and fears as soon as they arise.

Early warning signs can often lead to a proactive approach to care that may ultimately reduce the risk of injury due to increasing limitation.

Transportation Options

In spite of personal determination, exercises that maintain flexibility, or refresher courses designed specifically for seniors, there may come a time when driving is not an option. As you and your parent begin discussions about driving and the possibility of giving it up one day, you will want to explore alternative resources available within your parent's community.

One option, enjoyed by many seniors is the motorized scooter. There are a variety of these on the market today and each is designed to appeal to specific requirements and self-image of the users. Being able to run errands, carry parcels, or simply visit areas beyond walking distance is very appealing to someone who has been used to the independence afforded by driving. Like all mobility aids, it is important that a scooter 'fit' the user. It should be neither too small nor too large or heavy for the driver to handle. Like any new experience, allowance must be made for practice sessions and even a good deal of trial and error in a safe location as your parent adjusts, not only to the feel, the balance, and the driving mechanics, but to sharing a sidewalk as well. Even the most courteous driver has to learn a new set of 'manners' when driving on the sidewalk.

While it allows a degree of mobility and independence, many of the concerns about compromised driving are relevant to scooters drivers. Failing eyesight, reduced hearing ability and diminished flexibility are valid reasons to forego the purchase of a motorized vehicle. These limitations could severely compromise the safety of the driver as well as pedestrians sharing the same sidewalk. One of the frustrations and biases expressed toward seniors arises from the lack of courtesy and potential physical contact with scooter drivers on city sidewalks. While these incidents may reflect the attitudes of a few, they reinforce the need for caution.

If the decision is made that self-driven motorized transportation is not appropriate for your parent, you will want to explore public and/or private modes of transportation. In an earlier section we have discussed scheduling the regular delivery of prescription medicine and groceries as well as organizing standing appointments for in-home personal services, however, there are many times when we must or want to travel outside our immediate environment.

Medical Transport

Obviously the local ambulance service will respond to emergency medical issues. However, there are other public or private medical transport services that can be scheduled for transport to a variety of appointments and events. In some cases, the attendant will accompany the patient to the appointment and return them to their home/room safely. Stretchers are available in most vehicles. However, if the client is able to sit, portal to portal wheel chair service is provided. The patient may, unless otherwise necessary during a medical examination, remain in the wheel chair throughout the process. You may want to explore these services, associated costs, scheduling details and billing arrangements before the services are required. Understanding ahead of time, that this option is available, may help to ease any confusion or uncertainty around a new experience.

Public Transport

Most urban areas offer discounted transit service for seniors. Providing your parent is fit and aware enough to follow schedules and directions, knows where s/he is going and how they are returning, and are able to manage getting on and off public transit, the bus offers a viable alternative to driving. A major consideration, however, is the issue of travelling alone in less familiar, high traffic or unsavory areas. If your parent is used to driving alone outside his/her immediate area, they may adapt to the bus more easily than someone who rarely, if ever, drove alone or ventured far beyond home. Still, it may be prudent for you or another family member to accompany your parent on regular bus rides until s/he is comfortable following the procedure on their own.

Some transit companies also run a call-for-service bus that is designed to support disabled or limited-mobility clients. In some communities, the transit system works in partnership with a taxi company that offers discount coupons for seniors. These are requested when coupons or passes are ordered for the public transit on-call service. It is wise to see if this option would work for your parent before such services become necessary, as there is paperwork required ahead of time and discount passes and/or taxi coupons are often mailed.

Even smaller communities tend to have a reputable taxi service which responds to calls for service, and drivers will often assist elderly passengers to the door of their destination. Always check payment options before you need this service. Some companies offer their own credit cards to registered clients; others will accept most major credit cards. Often a monthly invoice works better for some passengers than the necessity of carrying correct change. Even in major cities, however, there are some taxi companies that will only accept cash. It is always best to check with the company before using their services.

Private Shuttles

Selected shopping or other commercial ventures offer a complimentary shuttle service to patrons wishing to avoid driving or parking issues. As well, very developed communities may offer regularly scheduled shuttle service that follows a well defined route covering shopping, banking, medical, restaurant and recreation-focused businesses in the area. If your parent lives in such a community, you may want to explore the possibility of this service as an option to driving, even if s/he still retains a driving license. In most cases, these shuttles are a free and effective way to ease into dependence on public transportation.

The work sheet at the end of this section is offered as a guide to help you collect the information necessary to explore the various alternative transportation options. Having this information as you address the issue of driving with your parent may lessen the shock or confusion around the possibility of not being able to drive.

Independence is a very precious commodity. Most of us are unwilling to give it up. Knowing that there are options to help us extend it often lessens the sense of loss. Working through these options with someone s/he trusts helps to reinforce that your parent is not facing this significant change alone.

Record of Physical Activity

RECORD OF PHYSICAL ACTIVITY©

Date_____

Physical Activity	Self	Group	Support Required
Walking/Running			
Aerobics/Gym			
Yoga/Tai Chi			
Dancing			
Cards/Games			
Sports			
Golf			
Skating			
Curling			
Fishing			
Darts			
Ping Pong			
Badminton/Tennis			
Bowling/Bocce			
Horseshoes			
Shuffleboard			
Rowing/Paddling			
Swimming			
Crafts			
Knitting/Crocheting			
Sewing/Quilting			
Wood/Metal Working			
Arts			
Painting			
Photography			
Writing/Poetry			
Scrapbooking			
Musical Instruments			
Other			

Transportation Options Sheet

TRANSPORTATION OPTIONS

Service	Contact Information	Notes
Emergency		
Ambulance (Option 1)		
Ambulance (Option 2)		
Non-Emergency		
Medi-Van (Option 1)		
Medi-Van (Option 2)		
Disability Bus (Option 1)		
Disability Bus (Option 2)		
Discount Taxi (Option 1)		
Discount Taxi (Option 2)		
Shuttle Service		
Other		

Health and Personal Care

In the midst of winter, I found in me an invincible summer.

Albert Camus

Life has a way of throwing curve balls at us just when we feel we have it all together. This uncertainty of what tomorrow holds increases with age. It is important, therefore, to have done some contingency, or in plainer language, some *'what-if'* thinking, so you're not caught off guard should your parent experience a setback. The following information is included to assist with the process of doing just that, thinking about the *'what-ifs'*.

What if your parent falls, faints, demonstrates a serious change in physical condition, or quite suddenly experiences significant loss of cognitive abilities. Are you aware of the symptoms of stroke or heart attack? Here is the U.S. Government summary of stroke symptoms:

1. Sudden numbness or weakness of the face, arm or leg, especially on one side of the body

137

2. Sudden confusion or problems understanding
3. Sudden difficulty speaking
4. Sudden vision difficulty in one or both eyes
5. Sudden dizziness, loss of balance or coordination, or difficulty walking
6. Sudden, severe headache with no apparent cause.

Health Canada lists the following symptoms for Heart Attack (Myocardial Infarction)

1. Shortness of breath
2. Anxiety
3. Sweating
4. Confusion
5. Nausea and vomiting
6. Temporary changes in vision
7. Light-headedness.

What are the chances that you would be with your parent should any of the above changes in his/her condition occur? If not you, then who?

Given the likelihood that you would not be first on the scene, you will want to ensure that information pertaining to your parent's well being is current and posted in clear view of attending medical personnel (the refrigerator door is ideal). The following information should be included:

- your parent's full name, birth date, Social Security/Insurance Numbers
- medical insurance and drug plan(s) numbers
- your parent's blood type, allergies, special needs/conditions
- how to contact your parent's physician/medical health practitioner
- your name, relationship, and emergency contact information
- the name and dose of each medication your parent takes
- the location of medication blister pack(s)
- name of hospital of choice – if you have a choice
- emergency transport options and numbers
- non-emergency transport options and numbers
- Do Not Resuscitate Order (if applicable)

Given the likelihood that you would not be first on the scene, you will want to ensure that information pertaining to your parent's well-being is current and posted in clear view of attending medical personnel (the refrigerator door is ideal). The following information should be included:

A sample Emergency Information Sheet is included at the end of this section; you may use this sheet as is, or adapt it to suit your specific needs. You may wish to check with the Emergency health authorities in your area to determine if they have developed an information sheet tailored to their response system. Some examples of pre-designed forms are provided through links in the resources section at the end of the book.

As well as being posted in a prominent location in your parent's home, your parent should carry this information in a wallet or purse at all times. Both must be kept up-to-date, and the wallet copies should be plastic laminated. You will need to keep a copy for yourself, as will other Powers of Attorney, emergency contacts, and external caregivers. You may want to keep this information, together with an original and copy of the current Power of Attorney, where you can grab it quickly when notified that your parent has been transported to hospital. You may also want a copy of this information in your car.

CAUTION: *If there are transport options in your area, you might want to include your preference with the posted information. That way, you can avoid heavy invoices from agencies not covered by your insurance. In a non-critical situation,* *you may want to have your parent transported to their physician via discounted taxi, public on-call medical transit service, or private medical transport. These options are considerably less expensive. However, if the physician determines that hospitalization is required, transport is generally via an ambulance.*

The Transportation Options Chart© at the end of the previous section will help you assemble details specific to each transport option. In the Note section, you may want to include those covered by your insurance, additional charges, contact information, general lead time between first call and scheduled appointment, and any other specifics relevant to transporting your parent in emergency and non-emergency situations.

As well as having pertinent information to assist emergency personnel in a crisis, you may want to help your parent put together their personal emergency kit to take with them to hospital. Apart from a spare toothbrush, toothpaste, comb/brush, hand cream, lip balm, and tissues, your parent may want travel size toiletries, a favorite magazine, a small clock, a notepad, a pen and a telephone directory with key numbers noted. You may also wish to have copies of current prescriptions, although the attending physician may alter the medications your parent requires. Finally, you will need a current copy of your parent's master calendar so you can postpone or cancel outstanding appointments and as well, a list of close friends and family who would want to know of any changes in your parent's status or routine. This info may already be on your mobile device. Finally, it is imperative that you familiarize yourself with the "Do Not Resuscitate (DNR) Order", an increasingly common method of managing the end of life process. Do Not Resuscitate Orders are outside the scope of this guide as they are legal documents and must be managed accordingly. It is important, however, to be aware that they are jurisdiction specific. Although they are generally similar, the details vary from State to State, and Province to Province. Examples of DNR's may be viewed on the sites referenced at the end of this Guide.

Medical Concerns

If reality alters suddenly or if behavior changes radically for no apparent reason, it is prudent to check out any physical concerns before accepting a diagnosis of potential mental/emotional disturbance. For example, bladder infections in the elderly can often trigger confusion, erratic reasoning or altered realities. Studies have shown that a regular drink of cranberry juice can lessen the chance of bladder infections. Be sure to check labels. While concentrated, organic, pure cranberry juice is quite effective, it has to be cut with five times the amount of water and is still rather bitter. Alternatively, it may be better (and a whole lot less expensive) to search out cranberry juice that is effective yet pleasant to take. Some people keep a supply of Cranberry extract tablets on hand to administer regularly or as required. Some of those sold through health food stores may even include probiotics to rebalance the flora of the gut.

Try to be objective when assessing changes in your parent's behavior. If a bath was a weekly occurrence it is perfectly natural for your parent to react negatively when daily showers/baths are encouraged. If, however, you begin to notice that reality slips away to be replaced with an urgent desire to be somewhere from the past, often distant past, it may be time to have your parent assessed professionally. Similarly, dramatic changes in behavior, daily routines, etc., may also trigger the need for professional assessment. In the section entitled 'When Independence Is Not Enough' you completed The Personal Care and Physical Activity Base Line Chart©. You may want to refer to this chart whenever you sense that your parent's behavior has altered. Be aware, however, that some of these changes may be caused by the environment. Some such triggers are listed below.

Sundowning

Characterized by increased agitation and confusion, Sundowning is a delirious state occurring in late afternoon or early evening. According to The Alzheimer Society, Sundowning seems to be related to a malfunction in the body's natural sleep-awake rhythms and may be related to the inability to deal with stress.

Potential Triggers of Sundowning:

- fatigue (mental and physical)
- disruption of sleep pattern
- hunger or thirst
- low lighting
- boredom
- over-stimulation.

To Help Prevent Sundowning:

- increase exposure to light at dusk or on dull days
- check eye glasses and hearing aids
- check basic needs: thirst, hunger, toileting, discomfort
- plan activities and exercise early in the day
- spend time outdoors if possible

- encourage afternoon naps
- monitor diet; restrict sweets and caffeine drinks to morning hours
- change sleeping arrangements; a nightlight might minimize agitation
- provide a routine
- provide a safe environment.

Dealing With Sundowning:

- comfort/reassure, remind him/her of the time, stay calm and avoid arguments
- distract with favorite object, activity, or soft music
- reduce stimulation such as TV or radio, talk softly, ask visitors to leave
- seek medical advice.

Wandering

Whether your parent is living with family, independently or in a full-care facility, it is important to ensure that every precaution has been taken to ensure that s/he is safe. However, approximately 60% of people with Alzheimer's disease wander away from their caregivers at some time during their illness, causing stress and anxiety for the caregiver(s) and for the person with dementia.

There are several possible reasons for wandering:

- searching for the past; rather than correcting what is being said, focus on what the person is feeling rather than the accuracy of what they say
- continuing a habit or routine such as heading for work
- relieving boredom, seeking fulfillment, need to keep mentally busy or physically active
- relieving pain/discomfort; check to see if all needs are met, if they are in pain, could the need to walk be a side effect of medication
- responding to anxieties; remove triggers from the environment; encourage them to talk about their anxieties and reassure them
- disorientation; familiar objects and pictures help give a sense of security
- memory loss; choose your words carefully as the last word heard is often the focus; extreme anxiety will require much reassurance.

Post-it notes may help clarify some confusion although there may be no trigger or reason why the person has chosen to wander. In spite of precautions taken to prevent your parent from wandering away from home or from his/her caregiver, it may happen. It is crucial that your parent carry ID at all times. In most cities, it is possible to register for a Safely Home bracelet with a local branch of the Alzheimer Society. Always keep current photographs of your parent; one a close-up face shot, and the other a full length body shot to assist the search and rescue process. As well you may want to prepare a list of likely wandering places.

Loss of Memory

Memory is an integral part of who we are and where we have come from. It helps us build and maintain our identity and the identities of those around us. It allows us to form impressions and perceptions and lets us know whether we are in a familiar, safe place. Memory loss is distressing for the person with dementia, the caregiver(s) and those in the immediate environment. It can be one of the earliest signs of Alzheimer's disease and interferes with the process of recalling names and faces, remembering recent events, finding misplaced objects, and may impede our ability to use language. As with so many diseases, early assessment and treatment may help to slow the progression and limit deterioration.

Emergency Information Sheet*

Section A.

Primary Contact Information

*First Name*_____ *Last Name*_____

*Street Address*_____

Apartment No _____

*City*_____ *Zip/Postal Code*_____

*Home Phone*_____ *Mobile*_____

Gender Male ☐   Female ☐

*Age*_____ *Birth date* _____/_____/_____

*Blood Type*_____   *Day / Month / Year*

*Primary language*_____

Do Not Resuscitate Order (If Applicable): Must be Attached to this Form.

Section B

Emergency Contact Information

*PRIMARY Contact Name*_____

Main Phone Number _____

*Business or Mobile*_____

*Relationship (son, daughter, spouse, caregiver)*_____

*SECONDARY Contact Name*_____

*Main Phone Number*_____

*Business or Mobile*_____

*Relationship (son, daughter, spouse, caregiver)*_____

*ALTERNATIVE Contact Name*_____

*Main Phone Number*_____

*Business or Mobile*_____

*Relationship (son, daughter, spouse, caregiver)*_____

Section C
Essential Medical History

Angina ☐   **Asthmatic** ☐   **Alzheimer's (Diagnosed)** ☐

Cardiac ☐   **Congestive Heart Failure** ☐

Heart Attack history ☐   **Bronchitis** ☐   **Emphysema** ☐

Diabetes ☐   **Dementia** ☐

Dialysis ☐   **Hypertension** ☐

Cancer(s) ☐ **(specify type and location)**_____

Seizure(s) ☐   **Stroke(s)** ☐   **TIA** ☐

Section D
Essential Medication List

1)_____   2)_____
3)_____   4)_____
5)_____   6)_____
7)_____   8)_____
9)_____   10)_____
11)_____   12)_____

Section E
Known Allergies

1)_____   2)_____
3)_____   4)_____

5)_____ **6)**_____

7) <u>None Known</u>

<u>Section F</u>

<u>Insurance Information</u>

Public Health Insurance   *Yes*☐   *No*☐
If <u>Yes</u> insert Plan Number _____

Do Veterans Benefits Apply?   *Yes*☐   *No*☐
If <u>Yes</u> insert Plan Number _____

Private Health Insurance   *Yes*☐   *No*☐
*If <u>Yes</u> insert Policy Number*_____
*Carrier Name*_____

Insert Current Full Body Photograph Here	Insert Current Head Shot Photograph Here

*Attach this form to a prominent, highly visible surface such as the refrigerator door.

Care for the Caregiver

I've learned that people will forget what you said, people will forget what you did, but people never forget how you made them feel.

Maya Angelou

As your parent ages you may want to create a supportive infrastructure within which you and your parent address and manage potential physical and/or mental limitations in an ongoing manner. Such an infrastructure may be as informal or casual as regular phone contact or it may extend to include scheduled visits from family, friends and/or professional service providers. Ultimately, it may be necessary to enlist the support and continuous monitoring offered within a residential care facility. However, until then, there are several ways to support both your parent and yourself with temporary respite care.

The Family Caregiver

It can be a frustrating worry when an aging parent chooses to continue to live independently. However, with an appropriate system in place, both you and your parent can relax, knowing that someone (it may often be you) is checking on their safety and well-being.

Often the role of family caregiver is not chosen. It can be as simple as geographical proximity; you live closest to your parent or your parent has chosen to live with you. Position in the family unit also may play a role, as may gender. The eldest daughter, for instance, may often assume responsibility for Mom or Dad. Whatever the cause, the role of family caregiver may have fallen to you.

Respite Care

Much of this book has been dedicated to physical and emotional ways you can help your parent maintain their independence or choose an alternative lifestyle when that is no longer possible. This section is designed to offer respite care suggestions that may help you take care of yourself, while ensuring your parent's continued happiness and well-being.

By nature, most family caregivers focus on caring for others and often neglect their own need for rest and support. Respite Care, short-term or emergency senior care in the absence of a primary or family caregiver, is available in a variety of in-home, adult day-care, or short-stay programs. It is important to identify and utilize the variety of respite care options that are available to you. Some can be as simple as helping establish a *Buddy System*, whereby friends of your parent contact one another on a daily basis, checking to ensure that a 'buddy' has returned safely from an appointment, hasn't fallen during the day, has taken prescribed medications, and is generally doing well. The *Buddy System* works particularly well, if friends live in the same apartment complex or neighborhood. Such interactions are usually based on give and take.

CAUTION: *It is important to ensure that the interactions within these relationships are fairly balanced. Some folks may be used to someone supporting them, a spouse, an adult child, or a close friend, who is no longer available. In a reciprocal arrangement, it is important for both parties to guard against an imbalance. Taking advantage of a neighbor, friend or family member's good will could lead to an unhealthy dependence in one person and breed resentment and even hostility in the other. It is best to work* *out a schedule that clearly specifies who calls whom and when.*

Another respite care option, offered in many communities, is the Adult Day-Care or Senior Center. Located off-site, these facilities offer scheduled daily programs at least five days a week although, some may be open during the weekend as well. Generally, transportation to/from these activities is the responsibility of the participant or his/her family. There are, however, some Adult Day-Care facilities attached to full-care homes that provide mini-bus day trips. These may also offer a pick-up and drop-off service to regular day-care members.

In-Home Services

There may come a time, however, when mental or physical limitations preclude such arrangements and it is time to move to more at-home care. You will want to discuss the identified need(s) with your parent and listen to their comments and suggestions. There are many agencies or individuals that provide comprehensive levels of care. Some are based on user pay, with others care is determined by income and financial situation. Still others may function with volunteers coordinated through community, social or other non-profit organizations. It may help if you have prepared a list of local care options, the costs and any other specific information to respond to your parent's questions. A Respite Care Options Sheet© is included at the end of this section to assist you with identifying appropriate care options.

In-home services can be provided by volunteer or paid help, occasionally or on a regular basis. Services may last from a few hours to overnight, and may be arranged directly or through an agency. This option would enable your parent to remain in their own environment.

Stimulation, recreation, and companionship can also be provided by family members, friends or neighbors while you take a break. Community, faith or culturally-based and other non-profit organizations often recruit volunteers, while home-care businesses provide qualified staff to cover short, in-home intervals.

Various cultures prefer to have aging relatives live with family, either in a separate on-site apartment or as a totally integrated member of the family. Medical or personal care may be hired to address specific needs, generally offered in-home. However, the activities associated with daily living generally become the responsibility of the family.

In other situations, one or more members of the family assume the responsibility of regularly checking on the parent. In families that live close to each other, there are opportunities to create a phone/visit rotation system that effectively allows the various responsibilities to be shared. This can work by dividing up responsibilities among family members, assuming all responsibility on a month by month basis, or however it fits best into the established routines of the family.

External Resources

Regardless of the choices made to ensure your parent is safe and well, there may come a time when the 'informal' services of family caregiver(s) and/or 'drop-in' resources are not available or appropriate. In fact, it is important for regular family caregivers to take extended time away from these responsibilities and seek respite care to bridge the gap.

Many communities offer a variety of respite care options. You may wish to discuss this with your parent's doctor or other medical practitioner. S/he may have experience with some of these options and could help you decide which would be most appropriate for your parent at this time.

Your local retirement homes, private and public residential care providers and even some hospitals may offer time-limited respite stays depending on your parent's medical and physical needs and on appropriate space and availability.

Again the Respite Care information sheet is included to assist you in assembling pertinent information well ahead of when you might need it. You may want to include any tax implication(s) inherent in each choice. In any case, choosing the kind of respite care that is right for your parent and for you is money well spent. You will return to caring for your parent refreshed and hopefully relaxed. It can be a win-win for both of you as you and your parent share the experiences you had while apart. As well, a short stay in respite care will often facilitate the transition in to a full time retirement or assisted living facility.

CAUTION: *Let go of any guilt you feel for leaving your parent at home. You deserve time away, even if just for a cup of coffee with a friend. It is essential to your physical and mental well-being and for that of your immediate family. Resentment can be a very invasive and destructive emotion. You will know when it's time to take a break.*

Respite Care helps prevent burnout and allows those who take care of family members to continue to do so for as long as possible. It provides opportunities for rest, relaxation, running errands or taking a much needed vacation. Prepare your list of options now. Check them out and be ready

157

should an opportunity present itself or your body is telling you it's time for a break.

Care of External Caregivers

As discussed earlier, there are many external care options available to you and your parent. Whether you go with an individual or an organization under which many caregivers work, you and your parent will begin to develop an ongoing relationship with one or more regular caregivers. It is important to nurture and support this relationship by encouraging the:

1. identification and understanding of responsibilities and expectations,
2. establishment and maintenance of an open channel of communication,
3. implementation of appropriate monitoring system(s).

You may wish to formalize these points in a written agreement, signed by both the caregiver(s) and your parent. It reinforces their understanding and commitment to the agreements if either you or another family member signs as witness. Then, should your parent want to minimize or increase the services rendered or you sense the caregiver isn't fulfilling the agreement, you can take corrective action. Samples of such agreements can be found at the end of the Role Clarification© Section.

> **CAUTION:** *It is important for you to maintain a professional 'arms length' relationship with your parent's caregiver. Guard against the temptation to view him/her as a confident with whom you can share your/your parent's views and opinions. This is a person in your/your parent's employ, not a friend or ally interested in forming a close bond. It is wonderful if your parent feels comfortable and happy in the company of his/her caregiver and wishes to acknowledge special occasions with token gifts. However, care has to be taken to ensure that the boundaries set out in the agreement are intact if a business relationship is to survive.*

Care for the Caregiver (Respite Care Options)

CARE FOR THE CAREGIVER
Respite Care Options©

Option	Facility/Contact info	Duration	Costs	Notes
Community Services				
Adult Day Care				
Senior Centre				
Other				
Hospital				
Public				
Private				
Medical Clinic				
Public				
Private				
Retirement/Seniors Homes				
Public				
Private				

CARE FOR THE CAREGIVER
Respite Care Options©

Option	Facility/Contact Info	Duration	Costs	Notes
Buddies				
Friends				
Family				

161

A Final Word

There is a time for everything and a season for every activity under heaven: A time to be born and a time to die,...

Ecclesiastes 3.1, 2 NIV Study Bible

One day your parent will no longer be with you. As well as the loss of one of the most significant influences in your life, you will have lost a treasure trove of precious memories buried deep within the stories of who your parent was.

One of the consistent messages of this book has been to engage your parent in relevant conversation(s) as early as possible, while his/her mind is alert and abilities are unlimited.

Many of these conversations are not easily initiated, especially if your parent is actively engaged in activities that bring joy and fulfillment to their lives. This is the time, however, to begin the process of seeking information crucial to your parent's happiness and well being as s/he ages.

An informal, yet highly productive, way of beginning these ongoing discussions would be to

163

'interview' your parent. It's a great way to capture and preserve family history while experiencing events through your parent's eyes. You may wish to video these sessions. However, that is a personal choice and would depend on many factors, not the least of which is your parent's comfort level with sharing his/her life in front of a camera. Some may prefer a more informal, intimate or private interaction. Another option for sharing special memories is to spend time together re-visiting family photo albums.

However you choose to begin the process of listening to how your parent is feeling about aging, informal conversations about people and events that contributed to current perspectives and beliefs may easily evolve to reveal more personal and current concerns or fears.

Later in this section, there is a list of casual open-ended questions, the responses to which may help you build the story of your parent's life. You may wish to turn such responses into a memoir to share with other family members; thereby preserving family history and stories that otherwise may be lost.

You may wish to paraphrase these questions to focus your interactions with your parent. Interjecting these subjects appropriately into casual conversations may open opportunities for further discussions and, as well, increase your parent's comfort level with sharing personal information. Listen to what and how the story is being told. Your parent's reaction to events and people in the past may give you insight into his/her feelings about self, personal limitations, and/or how they feel about dependence on others. Understanding this information may help you to better address your parent's future challenges, limitations and needs.

Capturing the Memories

There are many benefits to recording family history. Apart from the enjoyment of hearing about your ancestors and how they chose to live their lives, you learn of their joys, their sorrows, and the courage they needed just to survive. Listening carefully, you may also gain tremendous insight into your parent's perceptions and beliefs by observing their reactions to the stories they are relating. It is these perceptions and beliefs that contributed significantly to the way you were raised.

Please consider these questions as suggestions only. Modify, paraphrase, change or omit them as best suits the conversation and situation. Use them as a puzzle background into which you place the pieces of information as they are disclosed. You may be amazed at the picture that takes shape as your parent begins to share his/her stories.   The final pictures are yours or more correctly, those of your parent.   These questions are offered only as a prompt or guide to help you.

1. What do you know about our family before you were born?
2. Where did they live? In what kind of house?
3. How did you interact with your parents or siblings?
4. What did you do for fun? What made you happy/sad?
5. How did your family celebrate holidays, birthdays, or special events?
6. Did you feel your family was rich or poor – why?
7. Where did you attend school? What were your favorite subjects?
8. Did you have special hobbies or interests as a child?
9. Who was the major influence in your life? How?
10. What were the major turning points in your life?
11. Are there any medical concerns in our family?
12. If you had one thing to say to future generations, what would it be?

There may be other questions you wish to ask; add them to your list or simply interject them into casual conversations. The important thing about this exercise is to do it now. Gather the information before it is lost or becomes muddled should physical or mental abilities begin to decrease. Memories fade and those we love pass away.

Before the time comes to say your final goodbye to your parent, it is important for you to understand, and have prepared for, your parent's final wishes. Knowing what is important to them, the decisions they have made, allows you to prearrange and potentially delegate a number of essential activities.

Find a quiet, peaceful moment to raise the issues around your parent's passing. This may be done in reference to the recent loss of a spouse or while discussing the passing of a friend or acquaintance. How was this handled? Is that what your parent would want? How did they feel during the service? The responses to these and other 'soft' questions will give you the opening into casually discussing their preferences and wishes.

Encourage your parent to talk about the rituals common to your culture and/or religious norms. Does s/he adhere to traditional processes or do they wish something different? Are there special people they want to be involved with their service? Is there favorite music or philosophies they would like to share with those left behind? How would they like to be remembered?

There are many ways to gather this information. Depending on circumstances, it may be an ongoing process or, if the moment seems right, a full discussion may take place. Information Sheets to record your parent's final wishes, as they are revealed, have been included at the end of this section. You may wish to have your parent communicate major decisions to other family members to ensure everyone understands his/her wishes.

Reputable funeral homes often provide a guide book that outlines the decisions required before and after the death of a close family member. As processes and restrictions may vary from jurisdiction to jurisdiction, you may want to ask your doctor, funeral director, religious council, lawyer and/or other appropriate contacts for information and guidance with your specific situation. Each should be able and willing to explain the process from their unique perspective.

If your parent wishes to be interred elsewhere, you will want to contact the airline for their requirements. The same is true for cemeteries, masonry, etc. Basically each step of the final process forms part of the bureaucracy around saying your final goodbye. Again, the Information

Sheets included here will help you to organize and record key information essential to this process, including pertinent details around pre-payments for a variety of services.

Care Homes generally ask for a written account of last arrangements in the event that you are not available at the end. If your parent lives in an apartment, condo, or retirement home, it may be prudent to ask the manager or director about facilities or staff available to residents' families wishing to hold a service or celebration of life in a common room or chapel. As well, community or service groups often offer similar facilities.

In previous sections, you will have noted the activities, clubs, community, service or religious groups with which your parent is affiliated. You may want to review this information as you pull together the final arrangements for your parent. You will also want to consider older friends and family members whose mobility may be limited when you organize a service or celebration of life. In some cases, with family and friends living considerable distance apart, it may be necessary to organize more than one event to include those who were closest to your parent during his/her life. Finally, you will want to compile a list of folks to be notified of your parent's passing. This is definitely a task that can be delegated to other family members.

However, it is prudent to have a master list to ensure that all friends and family have been notified.

It is never an easy time when a close family member passes. It can be an emotionally and physically challenging ordeal. It is important, therefore, to have as much of the essential detail already organized, agreed upon and, ideally, paid in-full. There is a significant difference between pre-planning your final arrangements and pre-paying them.

Pre-planning itemizes options available at the time and reflects today's costs associated with the choices made. However, a few years down the road those costs will have increased, key personnel may not be around to remember you, and your choices may not be available. In extreme cases, organizations may have changed ownership or even closed. Your pre-planned documents may have been lost and you will be forced to begin again.

Pre-paying for as many of the arrangements as possible guarantees that those services will be available when you need them. Life marches on and it may be that key players in your parent's final wishes are no longer available. However, by formalizing commitments ahead of time, you will significantly decrease the grief-induced anxiety and confusion that often accompany making such choices under pressure.

While your parent is obviously the focus of these final activities, you will want to be aware of the impact of the role(s) you and other family members are called upon to play. Take care to support yourself and those close to you. Allow yourself the time to grieve and celebrate the life that was your parent.

Savor time spent with him/her knowing that the gift of your time was the best gift you could ever give. Remember the good times and how, together, you survived the many challenges over the years. Be grateful that you had the opportunity to share this final journey with your loved one. Treasure the times spent together and enjoy the precious memories for years to come.

The Author's Final Thought

There is no end to this book as life continues to evolve and with it, the joys and concerns of caring for a special loved one. Take the time necessary to review the information sheets provided at the end of this and other sections of the book. Complete those relevant to you and your situation. Update details as necessary and refer to this information often, especially as you observe a decrease in your parent's abilities or notice behavioral changes.

You may want to keep this book as a record of the time spent gathering pertinent information about your parent and his/her reactions to the people and events that intertwined with his/her life. Savor the moments spent listening to your parent; their thoughts, their joys, their sorrows, and especially their wisdom. Hold tightly to the stories and insights that provide a glimpse into who and what has shaped you. Whatever you choose to do with this information, or how you decide use it, I trust it helps to bring you peace and joy as you continue to share this incredible journey with your loved one.

Final Arrangements – Memorial Services (1)

A FINAL WORD
FINAL ARRANGEMENTS
MEMORIAL SERVICES (1)

	Contact Info & Details	Responsibility	Fees	Date Paid
Funeral Parlour (1)				
Funeral Parlour (2)				
Crematorium (1)				
Crematorium (2)				
Urn/Casket				
Cemetery				
Site Marker				

Final Arrangements – Memorial Services (2)

A FINAL WORD
FINAL ARRANGEMENTS
MEMORIAL SERVICES (2)

	Contact Info & Details	Responsibility	Fees	Date Paid
Location(s)				
(1)				
(2)				
Speakers				
(1)				
(2)				
(3)				
Eulogy				
(1)				
(2)				

Final Arrangements – Memorial Services (3)

A FINAL WORD
FINAL ARRANGEMENTS
MEMORIAL SERVICES (3)

	Contact Info & Details	Responsibility	Fees	Date Paid
Pall Bearers				
(1)				
(2)				
(3)				
(4)				
(5)				
(6)				
Flowersa				
(1)				
(2)				
(3)				

Final Arrangements – Memorial Services (4)

A FINAL WORD
FINAL ARRANGEMENTS
MEMORIAL SERVICES (4)

	Contact Info & Details	Responsibility	Fees	Date Paid
Music				
(1)				
(2)				
(3)				
(4)				
Programs				
(1)				
(2)				
(3)				
(4)				
Notes				

Final Arrangements – Notifications (1)

A FINAL WORD
FINAL ARRANGEMENTS
NOTIFICATIONS (1)

	Contact Info & Details	Responsibility	Fees	Date Notified
FINANCIAL INSTITUTIONS				
Bank				
Credit Union				
Life Insurance Carrier				
Investment Brokers				
GOVERNMENT AGENCIES				
U.S. Social Security Administration				
U.S. Internal Revenue Service				
Canada Pension Plan				
Old Age Security				
Canada Customs and Revenue Services				

Final Arrangements – Notifications (2)

A FINAL WORD
FINAL ARRANGEMENTS
NOTIFICATIONS (2)

	Contact Info & Details	Responsibility	Fees	Date Notified
Regular Mail/Deliveries				
Professional Newsletters				
Newspapers				
Magazines				
Business Associates				

Final Arrangements – Notifications (3)

A FINAL WORD

FINAL ARRANGEMENTS

NOTIFICATIONS (3)

	Contact Info & Details	Responsibility	Fees	Date Notified
MEDICAL PROFESSIONALS				
Physician				
Pharmacist				
Chiropractor				
Dentist				
Massage Therapist				
Caregiver(s)				
Other				

Final Arrangements – Notifications (4)

A FINAL WORD
FINAL ARRANGEMENTS
NOTIFICATIONS (4)

	Contact Info & Details	Responsibility	Fees	Date Notified
PERSONAL				
Family				
Friends				
Neighbors				

Final Arrangements – Notifications (5)

A FINAL WORD
FINAL ARRANGEMENTS
NOTIFICATIONS (5)

	Contact Info & Details	Responsibility	Fees	Date Notified
ACCOMMODATION				
Residences				
1				
2				
3				
Landlord				
1				
2				
3				
Other				
1				
2				
3				

Final Arrangements – Receptions

A FINAL WORD
FINAL ARRANGEMENTS
RECEPTIONS

	Contact Info & Details	Responsibility	Fees	Date Paid
Locations Options				
(1)				
(2)				
(3)				
Refreshments				
Gratuities				
Clean-up				

Credits

[1] Medically At Risk Drivers Centre

http://www.mard.ualberta.ca/en/SIMARDMD.aspx

[2] DemTect: a new, sensitive cognitive screening test to support the diagnosis of mild cognitive impairment and early dementia. Kalbe E, Kessler J, Calabrese P, Smith R, Passmore AP, Brand M, Bullock R

http://www.ncbi.nlm.nih.gov/pubmed/14758579

Resources

Emergency Medical Information Forms for the Elderly

Sample Forms may be located on the following sites.

Fire Department - Schaumburg, Illinois

http://www.ci.schaumburg.il.us/HHS/Senior/
Documents/EmergInfoFormWEB.pdf

Halton Region, Ontario

http://webaps.halton.ca/health/resources/
resource.cfm?ID=411

Emergency Medical Services, Toronto, Ontario

http://www.torontoems.ca/main-
site/pdf/ICE%20Sheet2012.pdf

City of Renton, Washington

http://www.mediconefoundation.org/wp-
content/uploads/VialofLIFE_editable.pdf

Do Not Resuscitate Forms*

DNR Form - State of California

http://www.emsa.ca.gov/pubs/pdf/dnrform.pdf

DNR Form - State of Florida

http://www.doh.state.fl.us/demo/trauma/dnro/ form1896.pdf

DNR Form - Province of Nova Scotia

http://www.gov.ns.ca/health/reports/pubs/PFEDH _DNR_form.pdf

DNR Form - Province of Ontario

http://www.forms.ssb.gov.on.ca/mbs/ssb/forms/ ssbforms.nsf/GetFileAttach/014-4519- 45~3/$File/TXT_4519-45E.htm

Seek out information about your own jurisdiction; rules vary from State-to-State and Province-to-Province

Notes

Notes

Notes

Notes